Forensic Psychiatry:
An Introductory Text

K L K Trick, MB, BS, MRCPsych, DPM
Deputy Medical Director, Consultant Psychiatrist
St Andrew's Hospital

T G Tennent, MA, DM, FRCPsych, DPM, Dip Criminol
Medical Director, Consultant Psychiatrist
St Andrew's Hospital

PITMAN

PITMAN BOOKS LIMITED
39 Parker Street, London WC2B 5PB

PITMAN PUBLISHING INC.
1020 Plain Street, Marshfield, Massachusetts

Associated Companies
Pitman Publishing Pty Ltd, Melbourne
Pitman Publishing New Zealand, Wellington
Copp Clark Pitman, Toronto

First published 1981

British Library Cataloguing in Publication Data
Trick, K. L. K.
  Forensic psychiatry
  1. Forensic psychiatry
  I. Title
  II. Tennent, T. G.
  614'.1   RA1151

ISBN 0-272-79637-9

Text set in 10/12 pt Linotron Plantin, printed and bound in Great Britain at The Pitman Press, Bath

FRENCHAY
HEALTH AUTHORITY
LIBRARY SERVICE

Forensic Psychiatry:
An Introductory Text

Contents

Acknowledgements

We would like to express our very grateful thanks to Mrs. Jean Cox for typing and re-typing the manuscript and to Mr. Norman Coates, Librarian at St. Andrew's Hospital for his repeated help in finding and checking references. Without their help the book would never have been finished.

1. Introduction

Forensic psychiatry forms part of the examination for Membership of the Royal College of Psychiatrists, yet relatively few psychiatrists gain any practical experience in this field before reaching senior registrar status. Indeed it is perfectly possible to be appointed a consultant psychiatrist with virtually no experience of Court appearances. Yet it is the lot of most psychiatrists working in areas that lack a specialist in forensic psychiatry, to be asked to give opinions in a whole range of legal cases.

Solicitors and barristers are increasingly expected to know when it is appropriate to ask for a psychiatric opinion, and having asked for it to know what to do with it. Such referrals may be initiated by a number of other agencies, such as the Probation Services, but very few members of these professions would lay claim to any specialised psychiatric knowledge.

There is considerable literature on topics of mutual interest to the trainee psychiatrist, the consultant 'out in the sticks' and the interested lawyer or social worker. This literature is not, however, readily available, and a considerable portion of it is of doubtful practical value.

This book sets out to provide an introductory text not a definitive academic treatise. It is hoped that the legal aspects will be of value to the psychiatrist, while the psychiatric aspects will be of help to the lawyer. No doubt each will find his own part grossly oversimplified.

In order to make it relatively easy reading, references in the body of the text have been kept to a minimum. At the end of each section a list of references for further reading is given, so that the interested reader can pursue a topic in greater depth.

The book is designed mainly to meet the needs of doctors studying for the membership examination of the Royal College of Psychiatrists. Nevertheless it is hoped that it will also be of value to lawyers, probation officers, social workers and all professionals whose work brings them into contact with offenders and the mentally disordered.

No attempt has been made to cover aspects of psychiatry and civil law such as divorce or compensation cases.

1

Part 1 Legal Aspects

2. The Legal System

English law is regarded as one of the major legal systems of the world, and has formed the basis of legal systems governing perhaps a third of the world's population. Law is not a static set of rules, but changes in response to changing circumstances. Much of English law arose out of the customs of the people and this persists as 'common law'. Increasingly, however, laws have been created by statute, that is as a result of Act/s passed by Parliament. The interpretation of both common law and statute law has been the responsibility of judges. When a particular judgement has been given in a case, and perhaps supported by the Appeal Court Judges, it forms a judicial precedent. In 1966 the then Lord Chancellor said 'the use of precedent is an indispensable foundation upon which to decide what is the law and its application to individual cases. It provides at least some degree of certainty upon which individuals can rely in the conduct of their affairs, as well as a basis for the orderly development of legal rules'.

Civil and criminal law

The law is broadly divisible into Civil Law and Criminal Law.

Civil law is concerned with the rights and obligations of individuals to each other. It covers such aspects as family law, law of succession, law of property, law of contract and law of tort. A tort is a civil wrong for which the remedy is a common law action for damages. It includes nuisance, negligence, defamation and trespass.

Criminal law is that part of the law which deals with acts which are considered to be offences against the State, not necessarily against an individual, and which are punishable by the State.

Criminal courts

The law is administered through various courts.

At the present time, criminal cases may be tried in the following courts:

(a) Magistrates' Courts
(b) Crown Courts
(c) The Court of Appeal (Criminal Division)
(d) The House of Lords

Magistrates' courts

Over 98% of all criminal prosecutions in England and Wales are dealt with by magistrates. In addition they deal with a great number of civil cases, and carry out administrative duties such as licensing matters.

Magistrates are laymen appointed by the Lord Chancellor on the recommendation of the Lord Lieutenant of the County. They undergo some basic training but are unpaid. They are advised on points of law by a Clerk to the Justices who must be either a barrister or a solicitor of at least five years' standing.

The function of a Magistrates' Court falls under two headings, a Court of Trial and a Court of Preliminary Investigation. Offences can be divided into three types:

(a) Indictable offences
(b) Offences triable summarily
(c) Indictable offences tried summarily in the Magistrates' Court if the accused so chooses.

In minor cases that are tried summarily, the defendant has no choice and the case is heard before at least two magistrates (except for some very trivial offences). In cases where the defendant, although entitled to opt for trial at Crown Court, decides to be tried summarily, the Magistrates may hear the case and if they find him guilty may either impose sentence then and there, or if they feel the crime merits a higher sentence than they can impose, they may refer it to Crown Court for sentencing. In these cases the Magistrates' Court acts as a Court of Trial.

In cases where the defendant opts for trial at Crown Court, the Magistrates sit to determine whether or not the prosecution have established a *prima facie* case. If they decide there is a case then they bind the defendant and the witnesses to attend the trial at a Crown Court. If the Magistrates feel that a *prima facie* case has not been made, they must order the release of the defendant. In these cases the Magistrates' Court acts as a Court of Preliminary Investigation.

Juvenile courts

Certain magistrates form a special panel to deal with offences committed by children and young persons. The Court comprises three lay magistrates, one of whom must be a woman. Proceedings in Juvenile Courts are less open to reporting than in the adult Court. Newspapers must not disclose the name of the defendant unless the Court gives specific permission.

Crown court

In all indictable cases (those carrying three months' imprisonment or more) the defendant is entitled to opt for trial by jury and the case will then be heard at the Crown Court. The Judge at Crown Court may be a Judge of the High Court, a Circuit Judge or a Recorder.

A HIGH COURT JUDGE is a puisne Judge of the Queen's Bench Division.

A CIRCUIT JUDGE is appointed by the Crown. He must be a barrister of ten years' standing or have held the post of Recorder for five years.

A RECORDER is a part-time judge appointed for a fixed term and prepared to serve on the Bench for at least one month each year. He may be a barrister or a solicitor of ten years' standing.

Offences are divided into four classes of seriousness.
1. Triable by High Court Judge only:

   (a) Treason
   (b) Murder
   (c) Offences under Sec. 1 Official Secrets Act. 1911
   (d) Incitement, an attempt or conspiracy to commit any of the above.

2. Triable only by High Court Judge, unless specifically released to be tried by a Circuit Judge, or Recorder:

(a) Manslaughter
(b) Infanticide
(c) Child murder
(d) Unlawful abortion
(e) Rape
(f) Unlawful sexual intercourse
(g) Sedition
(h) Mutiny or piracy
(i) Incitement, an attempt or conspiracy to commit any of the above.

3. Triable by High Court Judge, or a Circuit Judge or Recorder:
All indictable offences other than those above or in Class 4 (below).

4. Triable by High Court Judge, Circuit Judge or Recorder:

(a) Indictable offences which may be tried summarily before a Magistrates' Court.
(b) Causing death by reckless or dangerous driving
(c) Wounding or causing grievous bodily harm
(d) Burglary
(e) Robbery or assault with intent to rob
(f) Forgery
(g) Incitement, an attempt or conspiracy to commit the above offences.

House of Lords

This Court only hears cases referred from the Court of Appeal on the grounds that the case involves a point of law of general public importance.

3. The Relationship of Law and Psychiatry

The relevance of the mental state

There are those who regard all forms of criminal behaviour as being evidence of psychological disorder and thus consider that some form of psychological treatment is the appropriate management. Such ideas can be held both by those who believe that all behaviour is influenced by early childhood experiences as well as by those who feel that all human activities can be understood in terms of learning theory.

The majority of psychiatrists probably believe that such simplistic theories are not sufficient to account for all the vagaries of human conduct which they see in their daily practice. Exposure to the whole spectrum of human deviance may produce a conviction that nothing can be seen in black and white, only in varying degrees of grey. This attitude may make it extremely difficult for a psychiatrist to understand the way in which lawyers seem to try to reduce the most complex acts to simple logical events, each determined strictly by the event preceding it. Lawyers and psychiatrists often seem to suffer from the disadvantages of an apparently common language. They also suffer from the fact that most lawyers' ignorance of psychiatry is exceeded only by most psychiatrists' ignorance of the law.

The psychiatrists' role in relationship to the law has changed and expanded greatly in recent years. This has arisen in part because of advances within psychiatry, and in part because of changes within the law, both in attitudes and in legislation. The psychiatrist may be invited to give his opinion on the mental state of the accused for one or more of the following reasons:

(1) To determine whether or not the defendant is fit to plead.
(2) To determine whether at the time of committing the offence the accused was 'insane' within the meaning of the McNaughton Rules.*

* The spelling of McNaughton has been the subject of much debate. The form adopted here is that used in 'Daniel McNaughton' by D J West and A Walk.

(3) To determine whether the accused in a case of murder was suffering from such abnormality of mind as to entitle him to the defence of diminished responsibility.
(4) To determine whether there is evidence to support the defence of automatism.
(5) To determine whether the defendant, at the time of the crime, was capable of forming the necessary intent in those crimes where specific intent is necessary.
(6) To establish the presence of mental disorder which in the event of the accused being found guilty, might need to be taken into account in deciding sentence.

Before discussing these aspects, however, it is necessary to outline some fundamental legal concepts.

The aims of a penal system

The criminal law in Britain has evolved over many centuries, being influenced and modified by changing social and political conditions. It is not easy to define its aims and objectives which are often confused and sometimes contradictory. Nevertheless, it is possible to extract certain themes that seem to be important, if not always essential. The general objectives seem to be:

(1) To forbid and prevent conduct that causes, or is likely to cause, harm to individuals or to society in general.
(2) To define conduct which is regarded as an offence.
(3) To differentiate between serious and minor offences.
(4) To provide due warning that certain conduct is regarded as an offence.
(5) To protect the public from offenders.
(6) To provide official sanctions for such offences so that the offender is protected from unofficial retaliation.

The nature of the sanctions applied are influenced by the aims it is hoped will be achieved by their application.

Historically, the major purpose in imposing sanctions on an offender was to exact retribution, and that retribution should involve suffering on the part of the offender which was at least equal to the suffering of the victim of the offence. A system succinctly described in Exodus [Chapter XXI Verse 24]:

'Eye for Eye, Tooth for Tooth, Hand for Hand, Foot for Foot'

This retributive principle has been greatly modified by the more modern notion that the penal system should be concerned with the reformation of the wrongdoer. It has been advocated that such reform should be the main, if not the *only* object, in sentencing. This view does not seem to be held by many of the judiciary nor would it seem to attract widespread popular support.

The idea of extracting retribution from an offender carries with it the notion that the offender is blameworthy. In order to be worthy of blame the offender must be regarded as capable of exercising some degree of control over his behaviour and thus having a choice as to whether or not he commits the offence. Thus everyone, above a certain age, is assumed to be responsible for his own actions unless proved otherwise. It is in this respect that the mental state of the person at the time of committing an offence becomes an essential feature in determining his guilt.

Definition of a crime

The only lastingly accurate definition of a crime is 'an act which at the time it is performed is prosecuted by law'. The nature of the act, its morality or immorality, and its results may remain constant, but whether or not it is a crime depends on the state of law at that time: for example, if you killed yourself on the 2nd of August, 1961, you committed a crime, but if you delayed the act until the 3rd of August, 1961, you were just as dead, but no crime had been committed, thanks to the Suicide Act 1961 which came into force on that day.

Crime is of a public nature as against the private nature of civil law. In civil law only the injured party may sue. In criminal law any citizen may initiate a prosecution. Having initiated a private prosecution the individual cannot set it aside, nor if the case succeeds and a sentence is imposed can he pardon the offender. In civil law the person suing can terminate the case at any stage, and then, when damages have been awarded he can decline them and forgive the defendant.

Crimes are generally regarded as being morally wrong, yet it has been vigorously argued that enforcement of a code of private morality is not the function of the criminal law. Morality is only of concern when the immoral behaviour is so offensive or harmful to the public order, that it must be prevented in the interest of the community.

The elements of a crime

Before a man can be convicted of a crime, the prosecution must prove (a) that a certain event or a state of affairs which is forbidden by the criminal laws has been caused by his conduct and (b) that his conduct was accompanied by a prescribed state of mind.

The event, or state of affairs, is called the *actus reus* and the state of mind the *mens rea* of the crime.

Both these elements must be proved beyond 'reasonable doubt' by the prosecution.

If there is evidence of a defence, even though it has not been specifically raised by the accused, the judge must direct the jury to acquit unless they are satisfied that the defence has been disproved. There are many statutory exceptions to this rule. Where an onus of proof is put upon the defendant, he satisfies it if he proves his case on the **balance of probabilities**, and he need not prove it '**beyond reasonable doubt**'.

The principle that a man is not criminally liable for his conduct unless the prescribed state of mind is also present is frequently stated as:

'actus non facit reum nisi mens sit rea'

The mental element is usually referred to as the *mens rea*. *Mens rea* may exist without an *actus reus*, but without the *actus reus* there can be no crime.

Mens Rea

This is a technical term which is generally loosely translated as a 'guilty mind', thus implying a sense of guilt on the part of the perpetrator of the offence. No such emotion need be present for *mens rea* to exist. It covers the range of possible mental attitudes which the person may hold at the time of carrying out the action which constitutes the crime.

Firstly there is INTENTION. In this situation the person foresees the consequence of his action and desires it to occur.

Secondly there is RECKLESSNESS. In this situation the person, while not desiring the consequence, behaves in a way which involves taking a deliberate and unjustifiable risk that these consequences might arise.

Thirdly there is NEGLIGENCE. In this situation the person brings about a consequence by behaving in a way which a reasonable and prudent man would have foreseen and avoided.

Finally there is the situation in which the person behaves in a way which could not be predicted would lead to the consequences which occur. This is referred to as blameless inadvertence.

In most cases the intention, or recklessness, relate to the act that constitutes the crime. In some crimes, however, it is necessary to demonstrate an intent beyond the act that has been carried out. Thus a more complete definition of *mens rea* would be:

'Intention or recklessness with respect to all the consequences and circumstances of the accused's act which made up the criminal act, together with any other intent which the definition of the particular crime requires'.

The extent to which *mens rea* is required varies from crime to crime and will be considered under specific cases.

Insanity

Apart from being asked to speculate on the state of mind of the accused at the time he was reputed to have committed the offence, the psychiatrist may be asked to comment on the present mental state of the person awaiting trial.

It has long been a principle of English law that the defendant must be in a fit condition to defend himself.

Under the provisions of the 1959 Mental Health Act (Section 72 (1)), a person who is remanded in custody awaiting trial and is adjudged by two medical practitioners to be suffering from mental illness or severe subnormality, may be ordered by the Home Secretary to be detained in hospital.

The sanity of the defendant may also be brought into question when he is actually brought to trial. The legislation at present covering this situation is Section 4 of the Criminal Procedure (Insanity) Act 1964.

Fitness to plead

The fitness of the defendant to plead may be raised by the defence, the prosecution, or by the Judge himself. The question of fitness to plead is decided by a jury specially empanelled for the purpose. If the accused is found unfit then the Court makes an order that he be admitted to a hospital specified by the Home Secretary. He may be detained without limit of time, the power of discharge being limited to the Home Secretary.

It is possible that a person, entirely innocent of the crime with which he has been charged could thus be detained indefinitely without any opportunity to put forward his defence. Under Section 4 of the Criminal Procedure (Insanity) Act 1964, the Judge is now given discretion to postpone consideration of the accused's fitness to plead until the end of the prosecution's case. As a general rule, however, fitness to plead is determined as soon as it arises.

In determining fitness to plead, the following questions have to be answered:

(1) Can the defendant understand the nature of the charge?
(2) Can he understand the difference between a plea of guilty and one of not guilty?
(3) Can he instruct Counsel?
(4) Can he challenge jurors?
(5) Can he follow the evidence presented in Court?

It is obvious that in many cases the accused may be suffering from severe mental disorder and yet still be able to stand trial. Wherever possible it is desirable that the case be heard and the sentence determined by the Court. Though fit to plead, the defendant may still raise the defence of insanity at his trial. This is now rarely done as it was mainly used in murder cases when the death penalty was in force. With the abolition of the death penalty and the introduction of the concept of diminished responsibility in cases of murder, the defence of insanity is now hardly ever evoked. However, the legal criteria of responsibility still apply and it is necessary to consider these criteria for they remain the law, and also influence other defences such as automatism and diminished responsibility.

In the year 1800 James Hadfield attempted to kill King George III by firing a pistol at him. Hadfield had sustained severe head wounds in battle and shortly after had been discharged from the army as insane. He suffered from delusions and hallucinations 'imagining that he had constant intercourse with the Almighty Author of all things' according to his defending counsel. He stated that he had been ordered to carry out the assassination by God in order that his own life might then be sacrificed 'to save the world'.

The Judge hearing the case, stopped it saying 'if a man is in a deranged state of mind at the time, he is not criminally answerable for his acts'. The jury brought in a verdict of not guilty by virtue of insanity—which left the problem of what was to be done with him. The Judge, Lord Kenyon, said 'the prisoner for his own sake, and for the sake of society at large, must not be discharged', and remanded him back from whence he had come, 'in order to be dealt with according to the Law'. The Law at that time did not in fact exist, but on 28th July, 1800 an 'Act for the Safe Custody of Insane Persons Charged with Offences' (39.40 George III c94) received the Royal Assent with retrospective powers to order the detention of such a person in a place of safe custody, until His Majesty's pleasure be known. No specific places existed to meet this need and Hadfield was in due course sent to Bethlem Hospital.

In 1812 Mr Spencer Percival, the then Chancellor of the Exchequer, was shot and killed by a Liverpool merchant called Bellingham. Bellingham considered he had a grievance against the Government and having hid himself in the House of Commons, he proceeded to shoot the first MP who passed by.

This crime caused great public excitement and it is probable that there was some general feeling that it had been provoked by the lenience shown to Hadfield.

Only four days after the shooting Bellingham was brought to trial and such despatch hardly permitted an adequate defence to be prepared. The trial was a travesty of justice, Bellingham was found guilty and seven days after the crime had been committed he was executed. [2]

In 1840 a young man called Oxford tried to shoot Queen Victoria as she passed down Constitution Hill in an open carriage. There seemed no motive for the attack, and he made no attempt to escape. There was evidence of a history of mental disorder and the doctors who examined him subsequently were agreed that he was mad, though they disagreed as to the nature of his insanity.

The Judge, Chief Justice Denman, in his summing up to the jury said 'if a man were the agent of a controlling disease which he could not at all resist, he was not then held to be a guilty party, and he would be entitled to an acquittal on that ground'. Oxford was acquitted on the grounds of insanity.

On the 20th January, 1843 a Glaswegian wood-turner, Daniel McNaughton, shot and mortally wounded Edward Drummond, Private Secretary to Sir Robert Peel, the Prime Minister. He was brought to trial at the Old Bailey on 13th March, 1843.

It was clearly shown that McNaughton had for many years laboured under a number of delusions. He believed that he was being persecuted by a battalion of spies who followed him everywhere, threatening and abusing him. He had at various times gone to police officers and other public figures and asked for their help in ending his persecution. Gradually, the Tories became the focus of his delusional system and he determined to kill the leader of the Tory Party, Sir Robert Peel, the Prime Minister. In the event, he mistook the Prime Minister's Private Secretary for Sir Robert himself, and killed him in error.

McNaughton's defending Counsel Mr (later Sir) Alexander Cockburn, skilfully presented the defence of insanity and the case was stopped by the presiding judge after evidence had been given by various medical witnesses. Following his summing up, strongly suggesting that McNaughton should be found not guilty on the grounds of insanity, the jury brought in that verdict. In due course he was admitted to Bethlem Hospital by order of the Home Secretary. McNaughton's acquittal excited considerable public concern. Queen Victoria herself was obviously not amused and wrote to Sir Robert Peel:

> 'We have seen the trials of Oxford and McNaughton conducted by the ablest lawyers of the day—and they allow and advise the jury to pronounce the verdict of Not Guilty on account of Insanity when everybody is morally convinced that both malefactors were perfectly conscious and aware of what they did . . . could not the legislation lay down the rule which . . . Chief Justice Manfield did in the case of Bellingham and why could not the Judges be bound to interpret the Law in this and in no other sense in their charges to the juries?' [3]*

The matter was urgently debated in the House of Lords and it was resolved to ask the Judges to express their opinion as to the law of England on this topic. Five specific questions were formulated and a corporate act of answers were placed before the Lords on 19th June, 1843. One Judge, Mr Justice Maude, dissented from the general replies. The answers came to be called the 'McNaughton Rules' and have bedevilled this aspect of the Law ever since. In recent years the concept of diminished responsibility has somewhat lessened their importance—a development that Scottish Law had encompassed as early as 1867. The rules remain, however, the legal test of responsibility.

---

* Quotation from *The Letters of Queen Victoria* (Ed. A C Benson) by courtesy of John Murray (Publishers) Ltd.

The McNaughton Rules

The Rules may be summarised as follows:

1. Every person is presumed to be sane until the contrary is proved.
2. It is a defence to prove that at the time of committing the offence, the accused was suffering from a **defect of reason** from disease of the mind, as not to know the nature and the quality of his act, or (if he did know this) that what he was doing was wrong.
3. When a criminal act is committed by a man suffering from a delusion, then his responsibility is the same as if the facts with respect to which the delusion exists were real, e.g. if he believed that a man was attempting to kill him, and he killed that man, as he thought, in self defence, he would be exempt from punishment. However, if he merely believed that his victims had been responsible for his loss of wealth, or reputation, then he would be liable to punishment.

The Rules represented a considerable retreat from the humanitarian decisions made in the cases of Hadfield, Oxford and McNaughton. In most situations, the burden of proof lies on the prosecution, but the presumption of sanity creates an exception to this rule and places the onus of proof upon the defence.

The criticisms of the Rules were summarised by the Royal Commission on Capital Punishment 1949–53.

'The McNaughton test is based on an entirely obsolete and misleading conception of the nature of insanity, since insanity does not only, or primarily, affect the cognitive or intellectual faculties, but affects the whole personality of the patient, including both the will and the emotions. An insane person may, therefore, often know the nature and quality of his act and that it is wrong and forbidden by law, but yet commit it as a result of the mental disease. He may, for example, be overwhelmed by a sudden irresistible impulse; or he may regard his motives as standing higher than the sanctions of the law; or it may be that in the distorted world in which he lives, normal considerations may have little meaning or little value.'

When the accused is found not guilty by reason of insanity, he does not go free. He is ordered to be detained at the Queen's pleasure in a hospital to be selected by the Home Secretary. This is usually one of the Special Hospitals. The accused may thus be detained until the Home

Secretary is satisfied that he no longer represents a danger to the public. This is one reason why the defence of insanity is rarely pleaded.

In cases tried summarily in Magistrates' Courts the same defence can be raised, but the legislation regarding the disposal of the case is different. The Magistrates may allow the accused to go free if the defence is established, and there are no grounds for further action to protect society. Should such a need exist a hospital order may be made under Section 60 (2) of the Mental Health Act, 1959.

The rules and their interpretation continued to spread confusion among lawyers and psychiatrists until the defence of diminished responsibility was introduced in England by the Homicide Act 1957. Following this a defence of Insanity in terms of the McNaughton Rules is rarely embarked upon.

Diminished responsibility

This defence to the charge of murder, if sustained, entitles the accused not to be acquitted altogether, but to be found guilty only of manslaughter. It was derived from a defence in Scottish law which originated from a judicial decision of Lord Deas in 1867.

The Homicide Act 1957 (Section 2) states:

1. Where a person kills or is party to a killing of another, he shall not be convicted of murder if he was suffering from such abnormality of mind (whether arising from a condition of arrested or retarded development of mind or any inherent causes or induced by disease or injury) as substantially impaired his mental responsibility for his acts and omissions in doing or being party to the killing.
2. On a charge of murder it shall be for the defence to prove that the person charged is by virtue of this section not liable to be convicted of murder.
3. A person who but for this section would be liable, whether as a principal or as accessory, to be convicted of murder shall be liable instead to be convicted of manslaughter.

This gives the Judge a wide choice of punishment, including detention or compulsory treatment under the Mental Health Act 1959.

As with the defence of insanity, the burden of proof rests upon the accused and need only be established on a balance of reasonable probabilities and not 'beyond all reasonable doubt'.

Since the introduction of this defence, there has not been a marked increase in the number of persons avoiding conviction for murder on the basis of their mental disorder. The proportion of persons charged with murder who escape conviction on the grounds of mental disorder is much the same as it was before the Homicide Act came into force. It is possible that some who would previously have been found unfit to plead, and some who were acquitted on the grounds of insanity now plead diminished responsibility.

According to Lord Parker 'In order to satisfy the requirements of Section 2 (1) of the Homicide Act, 1957, the accused must show that (a) he was suffering from an abnormality of mind and (b) that such abnormality of mind (I) arose from a condition of arrested or retarded development of mind or any inherent causes or was induced by disease or injury and (II) was such as substantially impaired his mental responsibility for his acts in doing or being a party to the killing . . . [4]

Whether the accused was at the time of the killing suffering from any 'abnormality of mind' is a question for the jury. On this question medical evidence is no doubt of importance, but the jury are entitled to take into consideration all the evidence, including the acts or statements of the accused and his demeanour. They are not bound to accept the medical evidence if there is other material before them which, in their good judgement, conflicts with it and outweighs it.

The aetiology of the abnormality of mind does, however, seem to be a matter to be determined on expert evidence. Assuming that the jury are satisfied, on the balance of probabilities, that the accused was suffering from 'abnormality of mind' from one of the causes specified in the parenthesis of the subsection, the crucial question nevertheless arises: was the abnormality such as substantially impaired his mental responsibility for his acts in doing or being a party to the killing? This is a question of degree, and essentially one for the jury. Medical evidence is of course relevant, but the question involves a decision not merely as to whether there was some impairment of the mental responsibility of the accused but whether such impairment can properly be called 'substantial', a matter upon which juries may quite legitimately differ from doctors. The jury may decide that there is such impairment when the doctors say there is not and vice versa.

Automatism

It is generally considered that a person should not be held criminally responsible for an act over which he has no control. The degree of control that can be exercised is obviously related to the level of consciousness of the perpetrator of the act.

Some acts of violence have been committed when the person was apparently asleep, others have occurred during epileptic seizures. In both situations acquittal resulted.

If the automatism arises as a result of 'disease of the mind' then the defence is one of insanity and the onus of proof lies with the defence. What constitutes 'disease of the mind' is a question of law. The Law does not seem to be very clear as to what does or does not constitute 'disease of the mind'. In a case where a man suffering from cerebral atherosclerosis attacked his wife [5] the Judge ruled that the defence was insanity, but in the case of Charlston [6] who struck his child with a mallet and threw him out of the window, the defence that he was suffering from a cerebral tumour was regarded as 'non-insane automatism' which had to be disproved by the prosecution.

Automatism arising from psychomotor epilepsy has been regarded as insanity [7] while acts carried out during sleep, sleepwalking, hypoglycaemia and concussion have all been regarded as non-insane automatism.

In non-insane automatism the accused has only to introduce evidence from which it may be reasonably inferred that at the time of committing the act he was likely to be in a condition in which his ability to control his actions was impaired. Such evidence will depend heavily on medical reports.

According to Lord Denning [8] the defence of automatism is very limited. It can be evoked only in cases where the act was committed during unconsciousness or as a result of spasms, reflex actions and convulsions.

Amnesia

Obviously any act committed in a state of unconsciousness will not be remembered by the perpetrator. Acts carried out in states of altered consciousness may be only partly or inaccurately remembered. Events immediately preceding a head injury may not be recalled by the person suffering the injury.

In the case of Podola [9] it was argued that as a result of a head injury the accused had a total amnesia for the events with which he was charged. There was considerable medical argument as to whether he was suffering from organic, hysterical or feigned amnesia and in the event the jury took the view that it was not genuine and he stood trial. At appeal the Court held that even if the amnesia was genuine this was of itself no bar to his being tried.

Amnesia is thus not directly relevant to the question of fitness to plead. Its presence may, however, suggest the presence of some underlying disorder which itself would affect fitness to plead.

References

The relationship of law and psychiatry

1   West, D J and Walk, A (1977) *Daniel McNaughton, His Trial and the Aftermath*. Gaskell Books, published for the *British Journal of Psychiatry* by Headley Bros. Ltd., Ashford, Kent
2   Gillen, Mollie (1972) *Assassination of the Prime Minister*. Sidgwick & Jackson, London
3   Benson, A C (Ed) (1907) *The Letters of Queen Victoria*. John Murray, (Publishers) Ltd, London
4   R *v* Byrne (1960) 2 Q.B., 396
5   R *v* Kemp (1957) 1 Q.B., 399
6   R *v* Charlston (1955) 1 A.U.E.R., 859
7   Bratty *v* Attorney-General for Northern Ireland (1961) 3 A.U.E.R., 523
8   Gallagher *v* Attorney-General for Northern Ireland (1963) A.C., 349
9   R *v* Podola (1959) 3 W.L.R., 718

Further Reading

Smith, J C and Hogan, B (1973) *Criminal Law*, 3rd edition. Butterworth, London
Cross, R and Jones, P A (1976) *Introduction to Criminal Law*, 8th edition. Butterworth, London

4. Criminology

Criminology is a vague term simply meaning the study of crime and related phenomena. It is not in itself a discipline, such as psychology or sociology, but rather an area of study that draws upon several disciplines, namely law, sociology and psychology for its methodologies and theories. Any question one may wish to ask about crime, its prevalence, aetiology, treatment, etc., will therefore come within the general framework of criminology and may command different explanations, theories and ideas according to which discipline is examining the question. As yet no unifying inter-disciplinary theories for criminology exist.

Criminal statistics

Despite the considerable attention that has been drawn to the unreliability of criminal statistics they still form the basic data for many of the questions that criminologists try to answer. In this chapter, after a mention of some of the pitfalls and problems that one should be aware of in interpreting criminal statistics, some of the more relevant statistics relating to forensic psychiatry will be discussed, together with a comment on the psychiatric contribution to criminology.

Crime is only crime in as far as it is an act proscribed by the criminal laws of a country. As laws change so what constitutes crime changes. The frequency with which a crime appears in criminal statistics depends on how criminal laws are enforced. Societal pressures, local policing policy, and law enforcement directives play a part in the degree to which offences are both recorded or indeed investigated. Such changes can have very large effects on the apparent prevalence of given crimes over years and between countries.

Many crimes have to be reported to the police before they are officially known to exist, hence factors that affect the public's attitude to reporting crime will affect the recorded statistics. These attitudes may change or vary. Other crimes depend on police observation to be detected; thus areas which are heavily policed or where observation of behaviour is easier may have apparently higher crime rates. It is often argued that much of the differences in crime rates between social classes can be explained in terms of sociological differences rather than real differences in behaviour or criminality of the different groups. These are but a few of the factors that one must be aware of in interpreting criminal statistics.

Despite the pitfalls, criminal statistics remain an important part of criminology. Amongst other things they indicate that crime is associated with age. Seventeen is the peak age of offending. Longitudinal studies indicate that 7% of male children will have appeared in Court by the age of 14, and 15% by the age of 21. The life time expectancy of being convicted is 1 in 3 of the male population and 1 in 12 of the female population. Self report studies indicate that 90% of youths have committed indictable offences, so that committing an offence *per se* does not necessarily imply that an adolescent is abnormal. Property offences account for 80% of all offences, violent offences for 9% and sex offences for 3%. The psychiatrist, however, tends to see a biased sample of offenders and forensic clinics tend to see a far higher proportion of violent and sexual offenders. This tendency to see, in the less common and less easily understood crimes (e.g. arson, certain sex offences), some mental abnormality is a problem that the psychiatrist who does not see many offenders must be aware of.

The statistical relationship between crime and mental illness is a complex one because the two concepts are largely unrelated. On the gross level, criminals may be expected to have mental illness as frequently as anyone else and mentally ill people may commit crimes like anyone else. In neither case is there necessarily any relationship between crime and mental illness. On another level those who have had mental illness may be left so socially incapacitated by their illness that they drift into criminal behaviour. It would be difficult to argue that their mental illness had caused their criminal behaviour, but it undoubtedly can contribute to it. Matters are further complicated by the fact that most studies of the mental health of criminals (or indeed the criminal behaviour of the mentally ill) have been confined to studies of special groups, usually institutional groups and not the more general population from which they are derived. Among juveniles in the remand home setting, it has been estimated that approximately 15% show evidence of psychiatric disorder. Among Borstal boys Gibbens [1] estimated that 27% showed evidence of such disorders. For adult

Table 4.1

DIAGNOSIS	Admissions to:				
	Probation (Grunhut n = 484)	M.I. Hospital* (D.H.S.S.)	Hospital orders (Walker n = 642)	Special Hospital (Tennent n = 178)	Prison (Bluglass n = 300)
Schizophrenia	14%	13%	64%	60%	} 2%
Affective	13%	15%	11%	5%	
Neurosis	10%	16%	–	1%	2%
Organic	9%	4%	6%	4%	2%
Psychopathy	47%	20%	19%	29%	24%
Subnormality	7%	–	–	–	3%

*26% other psychiatric conditions including depression, not specified as neurotic or psychotic epilepsy, undiagnosed cases and admissions for other than psychiatric disorders.

populations Table 4.1 delineates the frequency of mental illness in different adult offender groups. These figures have to be set against the estimate of 14% of the general population who consult their doctors for psychiatric reasons.

Because crime is a statistically common phenomenon, it would not be surprising if many in-patients in psychiatric hospitals also had a criminal record. Figures are not available in this country, but in one study in the United States of America (of out-patients) 4% had a history of at least one serious offence.

Amongst the chronic destitute group there is a high correlation of commitals to prisons with commitals to psychiatric hospitals, and it is this group who need asylum in the broadest sense, who constitute a serious and currently neglected problem for society.

Some studies have also been carried out on patients leaving hospital. Early studies suggested that they were less likely to commit further offences than their non-hospitalised peers, but more recent U.S.A. studies indicate that they have a slightly higher expectation of conviction.

Organic psychological theories have had a long, if not entirely distinguished connection with criminology. For many centuries deformity and mental illness,were thought to be associated with criminality. Lombroso, the founder of modern criminology, based much of his theories of criminality on the physical configurations of criminals and this search for a relevant physical basis for criminality has continued. It has taken many different forms; somatotyping; the concept of a continuum of reproductive morbidity; and infective agencies: the last-named predominantly relating to the post-encephalitis syndrome (but recently reactivated to include other viral infections, e.g. herpes simplex virus). All these ideas reflect a similar basic interest in the organic substratum of behaviour, as indeed does the interest in epilepsy and criminal behaviour, in particular the relevance of temporal lobe disorder to disturbed behaviour. Genetic determinants of criminal behaviour have also been postulated, but more specific interest in recent years has focused on the possible relationship between sex chromosome disorders (in particular the XYY syndrome) and criminality. In all, however, the conclusions relating to any direct or specific relationships have been negative and any relationship has been attributable to intervening variables.

Psychological theories of behaviour

For many years psychological theories and in particular analytic based theories, dominated theoretical and treatment approaches to criminal behaviour. Delinquent behaviour has been seen as being equatable to the normal manifestations of the instinctive life of the small child. The preoccupation of delinquents with their desires and pleasures is equally manifest in the child; social adjustment has not taken place. This theory has had an enormous impact on workers in the field as did the early writings of Bowlby on the concept of critical periods of development, a theory renounced by Bowlby himself but which still finds its way into texts on development of human behaviour. More recently Eysenck's formulation of criminals as neurotic extroverts and Hare's proposition that primary psychopaths are high threshhold rapid habituates have revived interest in psychological theories of behaviour. For the practising forensic psychiatrist, however, it is convenient to have some working classification or framework within which to try and place the non-mentally ill offender and in particular the juvenile offender. Although over-simplistic, the classification proposed by Scott [2] has much merit, particularly as it attempts to relate a postulate of aetiology to a treatment approach.

Type 1
Trained but to anti-social standards—doing what is normal in their families or districts—not inconsistent with well formed 'character' or 'personality'. Their offences tend to be strictly goal motivated, the observer may well sympathise with the aims. Treatment required is retraining, i.e. to condition new behaviour.

Type 2
Reparative behaviour—intelligently, laboriously, often unconsciously worked out policy aimed at adjustment to society or to the personal handicaps which that environment has produced in him (e.g. inadequacy and inferiority).

The offender is identified with his pattern or misbehaviour and may even be proud of it. He is unlikely to feel guilty in relation to his offence, although he may feel so towards himself in other respects. The offence is goal motivated in gaining something for the offender in the emotional field. The trained observer readily understands and sympathises. Treatment should be aimed at trying to change the reparative pattern to one that does not conflict with the law. Some counselling is often required to get over the positive defence system which will be opposed to change.

Type 3
Untrained offenders—whereas the first two groups have learned effectively, if not wisely, these have not learned. They have no steady standards

of behaviour. The offender genuinely wishes he could resist impulses, but lacks ability to act with consistency—offences are goal directed but often rejected by others and are likely to be mixed in type. Behaviour is understandable in terms of weak personality and background. Treatment involves long term supervision with a background of sanctions—expectations should be kept low and attempts aimed to help the offender with problem solving in the hope that he will eventually learn this for himself. Heavy punishment is counter-productive.

Type 4
Rigid fixation—a very frustrating group to deal with. Here individuals tend to react or behave in a stereotyped non-adaptive, non-goal directed way, despite supervision. Punishment has little or no effect. Some behaviour appears to be actively seeking punishment, suggesting that punishment is anxiety relieving. Such offenders often dissociate themselves helplessly from their behaviour, the offence is often stereotyped and the individual seems to gain nothing apart from relief from immediate tensions. The observer tends to have little sympathy with the offender. The behaviour often appears compulsive but is not truly so for there is no element of resistance. Little is known about treatment but experience suggests that punishment is relatively useless. It may be that the 'therapeutic community' approach can help.

In reality, of course, most offenders overlap between these categories.

Female offenders

Until comparatively recently, crime was predominantly a masculine activity. Nine times as many men are convicted of offences as are women, and 33 men are sentenced to imprisonment for every woman so punished. This latter figure may well represent a chivalrous attitude on the part of the Courts. It is difficult to assess the contribution of 'psychiatric' illness to female criminality as the vast majority of women coming before the Courts are dealt with by fines and are not referred for psychiatric investigation. Only about 3% of women charged with offences are referred for medical examination.

Gibbens [3] studied women sent to Holloway Prison and found in both women who had been remanded for medical reports and those who had been sentenced to prison, a high incidence of both major physical and mental illness.

The most common female crime is shoplifting and the peak incidence is in the 50 to 60 age group. In this it differs from all other crimes.

Among women over the age of 21 who are sentenced or remanded to prison about 1 in 3 is, or has been, a prostitute. It would seem that prostitution is the female psychopath's equivalent of the male psychopath's criminality. Amongst this group there is a high incidence of alcoholism, drug abuse, suicide attempts and also of physical illness.

A crime usually thought of as being exclusive to females is child stealing. In fact the majority of people prosecuted for this offence are men. However, there has been no psychiatric study of male offenders. D'Orbán [4] has described 24 female 'child stealers' and divided the offences into three types:

(1) 'Comforting' offences
(2) Manipulative offences
(3) Impulsive psychotic offences

In comforting offences the woman steals the child in order to compensate for her feelings of loneliness and deprivation. Most such offenders have had disturbed family backgrounds, a previous history of delinquency and psychiatric treatment, and have shown evidence of personality disorder. The children taken were already known to the offender and were well cared for by her.

Manipulative offences were those committed in the hope that the partner with whom the woman was living would be influenced into remaining with her if he believed she had his child. The offence occurred at a time of personal crisis, often a miscarriage. The offences showed marked hysterical features in their personality.

Impulsive psychotic offences were usually committed by women with clear evidence of schizophrenia, though some were of subnormal intelligence and had transient paranoid psychoses. The offences were often bizarre and inexplicable, but sometimes were related to delusional ideas. A number of offenders had several children of their own who were in care, and had themselves been sterilised.

Walker [5] comments that 'in practice women offenders have a higher chance of being dealt with as mentally subnormal', and suggests that psychiatric diagnosis is influenced by the proposition that there is probably something abnormal about a woman criminal.

About 10% of women sent to prison are sent there for failure to pay fines. Many of these women are repeated drunkenness offenders and are, in fact, alcoholics.

In 1977, 105 women who committed indictable offences were made subject to Hospital Orders under Section 60 or 65 of the 1959 Mental Health Act, 32 for violent crimes, 37 for criminal damage, 11 for fraud and

3 for burglary. Five hundred and eighty seven men were similarly dealt with in the same year. Of the women 73 were regarded as being mentally ill, 15 were regarded as psychopathic and 14 as subnormal, the rest having either mental illness and psychopathy or mental illness plus subnormality.

In the ordinary psychiatric hospitals women outnumber men in the ratio of 1.4 to 1 but in the Special Hospitals men outnumber women by 4 to 1. Ratios vary with age: in the younger age groups there is an increasing tendency for female crime to increase, and in the upper age ranges the male/female difference is much less (3 to 1 in males over 40).

Felice and Offord [6] postulated two groups of girls who may drift into delinquency:

(a) Girls of average IQ from small middle class families with marked psychopathology in the parents.

(b) Girls of dull normal intelligence from poor families with three or four sibs; in 50% of cases the father is alcoholic.

Juvenile delinquency

The subject of juvenile delinquency merits a volume to itself. The majority of juvenile offenders who are referred for a psychiatric opinion are seen by consultants in child psychiatry or mental handicap.

The law as applied to juveniles differs from its application to adults in a number of ways. In general it is the concern of the Court to provide care for the juvenile rather than punishment (a trend which in some cases may soon be reversed).

The legal situation at present is as follows:

In law, any person under the age of 18 is an infant and in criminal law infants are divided into three groups:

(a) *Children under ten years*
Children who have not attained their tenth birthday are entirely exempt from criminal responsibility. If such a child commits an act which would be a crime if he were over ten, the only remedy at law is to bring 'care proceedings' in a Juvenile Court which may result in the child being sent to a Community Home.

(b) *Children over ten and under fourteen years*
Children in this age group are exempt from criminal responsibility unless it is proved that not only did they commit a criminal act but did so knowing it to be wrong either morally or legally.

(c) *Persons over fourteen but under seventeen years*
After attaining his fourteenth birthday, a young person is regarded as being responsible for his actions.

Anyone under the age of seventeen who is charged with an indictable offence is dealt with in a Juvenile Court, unless the charge is homicide, or where, if found guilty, he might be sentenced to be detained for a long period. After his seventeenth birthday he is regarded as being a fully responsible adult.

References

Criminology

1 Gibbens, T C N (1976) *Psychiatric Studies of Borstal Lads.* Maudsley Monograph No. 11
2 Scott, P D (1960) The treatment of psychopaths. *British Medical Journal,* **1,** 1641–1644
3 Gibbens, T C N (1971) Female offenders. *British Journal of Hospital Medicine,* **6,** 279–282
4 d'Orban, P T (1976) A typology of female offenders. *British Journal of Criminology,* **16,** 3, 275–281
5 Walker, N and McCabe, S (1973) *Crime and Insanity in England, vol. 2. New Solutions and New Problems.* Edinburgh University Press
6 Felice, M and Offord, D (1971) *Corrective Psychiatry and Journal of Social Therapy,* **17**(2), 15–33.

Further reading

Depression and Crime

Woddis, G M (1964) Depression and crime. *British Journal of Delinquency,* **v, iii,** 85–94
McCullock, J W and Prins, H A (1978) *Signs of Stress. The Social Problems of Psychological Illness.* Woburn Press, London
Neustatter, W L (1953) *Psychological Disorder and Crime.* Johnson Publications, London

Schizophrenia

Woddis, G M (1964) Clinical psychology and crime. *British Journal of Criminology,* **4,** 443–460
Kloek, L (1969) *The Mentally Abnormal Offender.* Churchill Livingstone, London (for A.B.A.)
Rollin, H (1969) *The Mentally Abnormal Offender and the Law.* Pergamon Press, Oxford

Part 2 Specific Offences

5. Crimes against the Person

Crimes of violence

Under the general heading of Offences against the Person are included a broad spectrum of crimes ranging from murder at one extreme to common assault at the other. The actual crime with which the offender is charged depends both on the severity of the harm done to the victim, and on the supposed intention of the offender. Thus if an offender sets out to kill his victim but actually fails physically to harm the victim, he may be charged with attempted murder. A man involved in a pub brawl hits another who strikes his head on the bar and dies—he is charged with manslaughter. Two youths beat up an elderly man, who but for skilled medical attention would have died, but because he survives they are charged with causing 'grievous bodily harm'.

Thus statistics based on the crimes 'as charged' are influenced by a number of chance and arbitrary factors. In considering the criminological and psychiatric aspects of violence other subdivisions are more useful than those of the criminal law. Recently particular interest has developed in the problem of violence within the family and this topic is dealt with separately (see below).

The matters of concern to the psychiatrist can be summarised as follows:

(1) What was the intention of the offender when he committed the act with which he is charged?
(2) Was this intention influenced by the presence of any mental disorder?
(3) Was he suffering from such abnormality of mind as substantially impaired his mental responsibility for his acts?
(4) If his offence was related to his mental state, what is the likelihood of him committing similar offences in the future? That is, how dangerous is he?

While these questions have to be considered in any case of violent crime, they are particularly important in cases of homicide and it is in this context that they will be considered.

Murder

The definition of murder
There is no statutory definition of murder. The crime of murder is the unlawful killing with malice aforethought, of a human being, by another person who is not insane within the McNaughton Rules, who is over ten years old and who is not suffering from diminished responsibility.

It is not murder to kill a child in the womb or during the process of being born, this being a separate offence.

The victim must die within a year and a day of the act in which the injuries were inflicted.

The Mens Rea *of murder*
The key phrase in the definition of murder as against other forms of unlawful killing is 'with malice aforethought'. This phrase has a rather 'Alice in Wonderland' quality as in law it does not mean what it would seem to mean in everyday language. The 'malice' may have nothing in it really malicious, and the 'forethought' need only precede the act by a split second.

'Malice aforethought' is not defined in statute, its meaning can only be derived from case law.

The Royal Commission on Capital Punishment said that malice aforethought:

'is simply a comprehensive name for a number of different mental attitudes which have been variously defined at different stages in the development of the law, the presence of any one of which in the accused has been held by th courts to render a homicide particularly heinous and therefore to make it murder'.

Precisely what these mental attitudes are remains uncertain, but they include:

(1)   An intention to kill any person.
(2)   An intention to cause grievous bodily harm to any person.
(3)   An intention to do any act, foreseeing that death or grievous bodily harm is the natural and probable result.

Manslaughter

All unlawful killings which do not amount to murder come under the heading of manslaughter. Manslaughter is generally divided into two main groups, 'voluntary' and 'involuntary'. In voluntary manslaughter, the defendant may have had the malice aforethought of murder, but there are some defined mitigating circumstances which reduce the crime to the less serious grade of manslaughter. These circumstances are:

(1)   PROVOCATION: Section 3 of the 1957 Homicide Act states: 'where on a charge of murder there is evidence on which the jury can find that the person charged was provoked (whether by things done or by things said or by both together) to lose his self control, the question whether the provocation was enough to make a reasonable man do as he did, shall be left to be determined by the jury; and in determining that question the jury shall take into account everything both done and said according to the effect which, in their opinion, would have on a reasonable man'.

(2)   DIMINISHED RESPONSIBILITY.

(3)   Where the defendant kills as part of a SUICIDE PACT.

Involuntary manslaughter includes all cases of unlawful killing where no malice aforethought exists. It includes causing death by gross negligence.

The distinction between murder and manslaughter hinges then on the intention of the perpetrator at the time of the act and his capacity to be responsible for his acts.

It is now rare for the defence of Insanity under the McNaughton Rules to be raised, and the defence of diminished responsibility is much more common. While it is only a defence in cases of murder, the same kind of arguments may be advanced as mitigation in cases of non-fatal offences.

The criminology of murder

As has already been stated, the difference between a fatal outcome of a violent incident may depend as much, if not more, on the skill of the doctors treating the victim as on the intention of the offender at the time of the offence. Separating murder from other serious woundings for statistical purposes may, therefore, give a distorted picture of the offender and victims. Within these limitations the picture that emerges (in England and Wales) is as follows:

(1) The majority of murders are committed by males.

(2) The majority of these males are aged between 20 and 30.

(3) Almost one third of murderers kill themselves before arrest. (These are mainly family murders and consist largely of cases in which children and/or the other spouse are killed by a parent.)

(4) Almost half of those charged with murder are found either to be insane or suffering from diminished responsibility.

(5) About a third of murderers have previous criminal convictions, about 3% having convictions for sexual crimes, a further 3% having convictions for both sexual and violent crimes, 10% having convictions for violent crimes alone and the remainder for crimes against property.

Refs: [1, 2, 3, 4, 5].

The victims

(1) Females outnumber males in a ratio of about 3 to 2, except in the case of children under the age of 16 where the numbers are about equal.

(2) About 75% of all child victims are killed by a parent or other older relative.

(3) Amost half the women victims are killed by their husbands, and most of the rest by relatives or close associates.

(4) Almost half the adult males are killed by strangers or casual acquaintances.

It is possible to divide murders into two broad categories:

1. Those in which the killing is committed by apparently normal people in whom no evidence of gross psychiatric disorder can be demonstrated.

2. Those in which the killer is found to have a degree of mental disorder such that he is found insane, or of diminished responsibility, or where he has prejudged the issue by committing suicide.

This second group is of primary concern to the psychiatrist.

Murder (psychiatric aspects)

Murder is not a single person activity, there must be at least one victim, and the interaction of killer and victim may be a much more complex business than the stereotype relationship of strong violent aggressor to feeble passive victim. No assessment of the offender can afford to ignore the role of the victim.

The mentally disordered killer

The mentally disordered killer may be considered under a number of sub-headings.

The psychotic killer

The psychotic killer is one who kills either because his awareness of reality is impaired to the extent that he is unaware of the nature of his action, or because his judgement as to the justification for his act is faulty. The former situation is very rare and almost always implies some disorder of consciousness at the time of the killing. It is thus almost exclusively related to cases of organic brain disorder.

R. v. Kemp (1956) (3 All E.R. 249)

This case is quoted, though in fact the charge was one of grievous bodily harm. The accused hit his wife over the head with a hammer for no apparent reason. He was shown to be suffering from cerebral atherosclerosis. It was argued that at the time of committing the act he was not aware of the nature of his act. The Judges ruled that cerebral atherosclerosis could lead to a disease of the mind in such a way as to temporarily or permanently cause a defect of its reasoning and understanding.

The second situation may arise as the result of any disorder in which delusional ideas or hallucinatory experiences occur. Probably the most common illness giving rise to murders of this type is severe depression, in which the sufferer develops delusions of hopelessness and decides that his family must be spared the horrors of life and kills them prior to committing suicide himself.

Schizophrenics sometimes kill as a result of hallucinatory instructions, but more commonly as a result of delusional ideas that the victim is in some way persecuting them.

R. v. Dadd

Dadd was a successful Victorian painter who developed schizophrenia. As a result of delusions of persecution he stabbed his father to death and fled to France. His intention was to assassinate the Emperor of Austria, but while travelling on a coach in France he stabbed a fellow passenger. At his trial he was found 'guilty but insane' and committed to Bethlem Hospital.

The condition of morbid jealousy which may be associated with alcoholism sometimes leads to serious physical attacks on the partner who is the subject of the delusional ideas of infidelity.

Rarely, people in mania, or hypomania, kill as a result of delusional ideas that they are entitled to do so as part of their exalted station in life. More often, such killings result from the irritability and physical overactivity of the hypomanic.

Patients with organic brain disease may also kill as the result of delusional notions in the setting of unimpaired consciousness.

It is important to remember that because a person is suffering from a psychotic illness before, during, or after a killing, it does not follow that the *act itself* was a result of, or was even influenced by, his mental disorder. It is necessary to establish a causal link between the two if the mental state is to form a defence and not merely a mitigating circumstance.

The sexual killer

A small number of murders are committed by people who derive sexual arousal from the actual act of killing, or by inflicting severe pain and suffering, which results in death. This is not the same as those who kill during or after rape, where sexual intercourse is the primary aim and the killing a secondary feature. This type of murder is considered in detail under sexual crimes (page 60).

R. v. Heath

Heath was charged with the murder of a Mrs Gardner who was found dead in a hotel in Notting Hill. She had been suffocated and prior to death had been beaten with a whip, her nipples bitten off and her genitalia lacerated. Heath had a history of multiple fraudulent crimes, and had on previous occasions inflicted wounds on sexual partners. He had also killed and mutilated another young woman. He was tried before the defence of diminished responsibility existed and was found guilty and hanged.

R. v. Byrne

This case was heard after the passing of the 1957 Homicide Act which introduced the concept of diminished responsibility.

Byrne killed and savagely mutilated a young woman in a YWCA hostel. The facts of the killing were not disputed and were admitted in a long statement by the accused. At his trial, three doctors gave uncontradicted evidence that he was a 'sexual psychopath, that he suffered from abnormality of mind, and that such abnormality arose from a condition of arrested or retarded development of mind or inherent causes'. He was found guilty of murder by the jury, but on appeal the verdict was changed to manslaughter—the sentence of life imprisonment being left unchanged.

The psychopathic killer
This group comprises most of those who are initially charged with murder, but who eventually are found guilty of manslaughter on the basis of diminished responsibility.

The concept of psychopathy and its relationship to crime is discussed separately. In this context it is used to cover a characteristic personality type, the diagnosis being based both on the recorded history of the individual's pattern of behaviour in all main areas of his life, and on his own statements regarding his feelings for, and attitudes to, other people.

In the terms of the 1959 Mental Health Act 'psychopathic disorder' means 'a persistent disorder or disability of mind (whether or not including subnormality of intelligence) which results in abnormally aggressive or seriously irresponsible conduct on the part of the patient, and requires or is susceptible to medical treatment'. Thus to justify the diagnosis, the history of the offender's life, apart from the crime with which he is charged, should show evidence of repetitive behaviour which is either damaging to himself in social and interpersonal terms, or which inflicts harm on those around him. Thus it is likely that his employment record will be poor; due to impulsive changes of job or involuntary dismissal following rows, absenteeism, drunkenness, or dishonesty. His personal relationships are likely to have been superficial and chaotic, showing his tendency to exploit people for his own gratification and discard them if they no longer satisfy him or start to make demands on him. There may be a history of alcohol abuse or involvement with other drug taking. There is likely to be evidence of previous criminal convictions, particularly involving violence or sexual offences. People who know him may describe his lack of control, his excessive response to minor frustrations and his apparent indifference to the needs and wishes of others.

The offender himself may describe his own difficulties in forming close relationships, his fear of rejection and his determination to 'get the boot in first'. He may also reveal his lack of concern and warmth of feelings by his expressed attitudes to the victim or the victim's relatives. His attitude to those responsible for his arrest, custody, defence and eventual sentencing may be all revealing.

Psychopaths may kill as part of a general pattern of violence, in which case the death may be an unintended result arising through loss of control, or because of factors in the victim making him less able to survive the injuries inflicted. Sometimes the excessive violence is provoked by unexpected resistance on the victim's part, though in other instances failure to fight back seems to be equally provoking.

It is not only the overtly aggressive psychopath who may kill. Megargee [6] described the 'overcontrolled' murderer. This is a man who for most of the time exercises an abnormally high level of control over his aggression, not responding even to high levels of provocation. It seems that being unable to disperse his aggressive feelings in small controlled amounts they build up until something triggers off an explosive response. After the aggressive act, he generally returns to his former rigidly controlled behaviour and may thus be the last person to be suspected of the crime. Such men may have equally inhibited sexual drives and the two facets may come together in repeated episodes of sexual killings.

In some cold affectionless psychopaths, normal emotional responses may be so diminished that killing has for them no special significance. Such men may become professional killers employed by organised crime, or by terrorist organisations as 'hit men', killing victims who have no personal connection with them.

The jealous killer
Morbid jealousy, which is discussed in a subsequent section, is sometimes the motive that drives the sufferer to kill the object of his possessiveness, or sometimes the person he suspects of having a liaison with her. It has been labelled the 'Othello Syndrome'. The sufferer becomes convinced of his partner's infidelity and starts seeking 'proof' that such activities are occurring. Thus he will examine articles of personal clothing and the bed clothes for evidence of seminal fluid. He may look for signs of illicit entry into the house or room and may set up

elaborate traps to reveal that windows have been opened to allow the entrance or egress of the lover. He follows and spies upon the victim, having often given overt encouragement for her to 'go out and enjoy herself'. Additionally he constantly taxes her with accusations of infidelity, often claiming that if she admits he will forgive and forget, saying that it is the uncertainty that causes him the most anxiety. Eventually, the partner may succumb to this pressure and falsely confess that she has indeed been unfaithful. Far from letting the matter drop this is often the point at which the accuser explodes into violence, justifying himself by quoting his victim's 'confession'. (In this description, the offender has been referred to as 'he' but the condition also occurs in females in whom it may also lead to murder.)

When examined, the majority of this group exhibit no other signs of psychiatric illness. In particular there are no other signs or symptoms of paranoid schizophrenia at the time of the examination. A small number do, however, subsequently develop such symptoms. A larger proportion are found to have alcoholic problems in addition to their paranoid symptoms, while the majority have some degree of sexual dysfunction.

The alcoholic killer
As mentioned above, some of those who kill as a result of morbid jealousy have evidence of alcoholism which may or may not be causally related to their delusional ideas. A high proportion of killings occur when the perpetrator is in some degree intoxicated with alcohol. Additionally it would seem that in about a third of cases the *victim* was intoxicated at the time of the event. (The relationship of alcohol to serious crime is discussed in chapter 15.)

Murder followed by suicide

West [7] studied 78 cases of murder followed by suicide. He found that the cohort differed from ordinary murderers in that there were a large number of women offenders and child victims and few offenders had previous convictions. The social characteristics of the group were similar to the general population whereas other murderers include a disproportionately high number of young unmarried males, and are drawn predominately from social class 5. He found that the prediction that most murder-suicides were committed by 'insane' persons was incorrect—only half the offenders clearly having mental disorders at the time of the crime. However, a substantial number were under considerable stress or suffering from physical illness when they committed the crime.

In a number of the cases in his study West found clear warnings of the impending tragedy had been given, but had been unrecognised or disregarded by various agencies. He emphasised the risk inherent in the case of potentially suicidal women who have small children.

The repeatedly aggressive offender

The majority of such offenders fall into the category of psychopaths and their violence is merely one face of multiple personality difficulties. A relatively high proportion of such people have abnormal electroencephalographs (EEG's). Hill and Watterson found that 48% of patients diagnosed as psychopathic had abnormal EEG's compared to 15% of the control group. On selecting those with aggressive behaviour the percentage rose to 65%. A study of apparently motiveless murderers by Stafford-Clark, showed a 70% incidence of EEG abnormalities.

The findings were consistent with the EEG of much younger people in whom they would be accepted as within the normal range. They included bilateral rhythmic theta activity in central and temporal lobes and episodic posterior temporal slow waves.

Williams [8] studies the EEG's of 333 men convicted of violent crimes. The group was sub-divided into those who had committed one isolated aggressive act, and those who had a history of repeated aggression; 65% of the latter had abnormal EEG's as compared to 24% of the former.

These and other findings have led to the postulating of a syndrome of 'episodic dyscontrol'. The majority of persons showing this syndrome are males with disturbed family backgrounds. They have a history of repeatedly responding violently to quite trivial stimuli, dating back to childhood or adolescence. Their outbursts of violence are sometimes preceded by an aura of some kind and may be followed by headache and drowsiness. Fifty per cent of this group have evidence of episodic changes in level of consciousness not associated with violence. They may be amnesic for the episode of violence and may express great remorse for their actions. A proportion show evidence of minor neurological deficits. Alcohol seems to increase the likelihood of attacks occurring, while phenytoin appeared to produce an improvement both in the frequency and severity of attacks.

References

Crimes against the person

1 1957 Homicide Act.
2 *Murder and Capital Punishment in England and Wales* (1974). National Campaign for Abolition of Capital Punishment, London
3 Home Office Statistical Department (1975) *Homicide in England and Wales 1967–1971.* HMSO
4 Home Office Research Unit Report (1961) *Murder.* HMSO
5 *Criminal Statistics in England and Wales 1977* (1979). HMSO
6 Megargee, E I (1966) *Uncontrolled and Overcontrolled Personality Type* in *Extreme Anti-social Aggression.* Psychology Monographs, 80 (5)
7 West, D J (1965) *Murder followed by Suicide.* Heinemann Educational, London
8 Williams, D (1969) Neural factors related to habitual aggression. *Brain,* **92,** 503–520

Further reading

Walker, N and McCabe, S (1968) *Crime and Insanity in England, vol. 1, The Historical Perspective.* Edinburgh University Press
Mowatt, R R (1966) *Morbid Jealousy and Murder.* International Library of Criminology
Parker, T (1970) *The Frying Pan (A Prison and its Prisoners).* Hutchinson, London
Myers, S A (1967) The child slayer. *Archives of General Psychiatry,* **17,** 211–213
Sayed, Z A, Lewis, S A and Brittain, R P (1969) An electroencephalographic and psychiatric study of thirty-two insane murderers. *British Journal of Psychiatry,* **115,** 1115–1124
Sallen, J, Meninger, K, Rosen, I and Mayman, M (1960) Murder without apparent motive. *American Journal of Psychiatry,* **117,** 48–53
Lackman, J and Cravens, J M (1969) The murderers—before and after. *Psychiatric Quarterly,* **43,** 1–11
Bruch, H (1967) Mass murder: the Wagner case. *American Journal of Psychiatry,* **124,** 693–698
Walshe-Breman, K S (1976) An analysis of homicide by young persons in England and Wales. *Acta psychiatrica et neurologica Scandinavica,* **54** (2), 92–98
Cole, K E, Fisher, G and Cole, S S (1968) Women who kill. *Archives of General Psychiatry,* **19,** 1–8
Cameron, J M (1973) Changing patterns in violence. *Medicine, Science and the Law,* **13** (4), 261–263

Hunter Gillies (1965) Murder in the West of Scotland. *British Journal of Psychiatry*, **111**, 1087–1094

May, A E (1968) An assessment of homicidal attitudes. *British Journal of Psychiatry*, **114**, 479–480

Brittain, R P (1970) The sadistic murderer. *Medicine, Science and the Law*, **10**, No. 4

Swigert, V L, Farrell, R A and Yoels, W C (1976) Sexual homicide: social, psychological and legal aspects. *Archives of Sexual Behaviour*, **5** (5), 391–401

Revitch, E (1965) Sex murder and the potential sex murderer. *Diseases of the Nervous System*, **26**, 640–646

Podolsky, E (1965) The jealous murderer. *Journal of Forensic Medicine*, **12** (1)

Driver, M V, West, I R and Faulk, M (1974) Clinical and EEG studies of prisoners charged with murder. *British Journal of Psychiatry*, **125**, 583–587

Resnick, P J (1969) Child murder by parents. *American Journal of Psychiatry*, **126**, 325–334

Resnick, P J (1970) A psychiatric review of neonaticide. *American Journal of Psychiatry*, **126**, 1414–1420

Scott, P D (1973) Parents who kill their children. *Medicine, Science and the Law*, **13** (2), 120–126

McKnight, C K, Moler, J W, Quinsey, R E and Erochko, J (1966) Matricide and mental illness. *Canadian Psychiatric Association Journal*, **11**, 99–105

Duncan, W J and Duncan, G M (1971) Murder in the family: a study of some homicidal adolescents. *American Journal of Psychiatry*, **127** (11), 1498–1502

McDermaid, G and Winkler, E G (1955) Psychopathology of infanticide. *Journal of Clinical and Experimental Psychopathology*, **xvi** (1), 22–41

6. Violence within the Family

While the incidence of non-fatal violent crimes has increased at an alarming rate, there are still more cases that do not come to police notice, and some which although notified to the police do not result in further action. These are cases of violence occurring at home between members of a family. In law, the offender will be charged under the various sections of the Offences against the Person Act depending on the severity and nature of the harm done without distinguishing between those offending against strangers and those who harm members of their own family. From the psychiatric point of view there has been increasing interest in intra-family violence, its managements and treatment. These areas of concern have been vividly called child battering, wife battering and granny bashing. There is increasing evidence of husband battering as an entity but this has not yet attracted a vocal pressure group to champion the battered male, and little so far is known about it.

There is obviously an overlap between individuals who use violence as part of their everyday technique of living, irrespective of their relationship to the victim, and those who are specifically violent towards members of their own family. There are, however, many people who only act violently within their own home. This violence may only be directed at the marital partner or it may also involve other members of the family. While it is convenient to consider the problem under separate headings, it should be remembered that violence to one member of the family may be part of a continuum of aggressive relationships. There is obviously also an overlap between non-fatal and fatal violence within the family, but the problems are not synonymous. Many of the killings result from a single violent episode, often as a result of a psychotic illness in the offender. The incidence of psychotic illness in those who batter their children or spouse is low.

A recurrent factor in all forms of intra-family violence is the contribution made by excessive drinking.

Parents who kill their children

The majority of women who kill, kill their own children, whereas of men who kill, only about 15% kill their own children. The overall proportion of male killers to female is about 4 to 1, so that in effect about the same number of men and women kill their children in a year.

There have been a number of attempts to classify the various types of child murder within the family on the basis of motivation or psycho-pathology. No attempt is wholly satisfactory; the following is modified from that suggested by Scott [1].

(1)　Mercy killing—where the child has a real source of suffering or handicap and where there is little secondary gain for the parents.

(2)　Psychotic killing—where the killing is a direct result of some demonstrable psychotic illness in the killer.

(3)　Killing as the end result of battering—in these cases there will be evidence of repeated assaults.

(4)　Killing in one explosive episode without previous evidence of battering.

　　In this type there are two sub-groups:

　　(a)　Those cases in which, as in child battering, the child itself acts as the stimulus by its behaviour.

　　(b)　Those cases in which the child is killed as a substitute for the person to whom the killer actually feels murderous.

(5)　Killing as part of sexual abuse or to silence a witness. Though this is a theoretical possibility it would seem to be almost unknown in parent/child murder.

(6)　Deliberate killing of an 'inconvenient' child

　　(a)　by assault

　　(b)　by neglect.

When divided up along these lines, some interesting differences emerge between the father as killer and the mother as killer.

Fathers

Almost half the victims killed by fathers fall into groups 3 and 6—that is cases where the child's behaviour is claimed by father to be the reason for the assault. About a third of the fathers are regarded as having some form of psychotic illness.

Mothers

About 90% of mothers who kill their children (excluding infanticide) are regarded as being psychotic at the time of the killing. This is supported to some extent by the greater incidence of suicide or suicidal attempts in women at the time of the killing. It may to some extent be exaggerated by the attitude that many hold that a mother who kills her offspring *must* be sick, while a father who does so must be a monster. The figures are also derived from cases dealt with before 'child battering' was widely recognised, and it is possible that some cases regarded as a 'one off' event, were in fact the end result of previous assaults.

Battering fathers who kill

Scott has also studied a series of fathers who killed as part of the battering syndrome [2]. He found that two-thirds of the men were not married to their partner and half of them were not the actual father of the child. Two-thirds of the fathers had previous convictions, about one-third having convictions for violent crimes. The majority were recorded as having a high level of personality disorder. Most had experienced parental violence in their own childhood though a few had not. A quarter of these fathers had reversed the 'work/child caring' role and were left at home with children not their own while their mother was at work.

A picture emerges of the sort of situation in which small children are at the greatest risk. That is as follows: a young man recently released from prison with a history suggestive of personality problems cohabits with a young woman who has living with her small children of a previous relationship. She is working full time while he is unemployed. The children as a result of previous experiences may be restless, tearful and mistrustful. The father regards the child as wilful or defiant, or sees it as a rival, and has totally unrealistic expectations of its behaviour, expecting it to respond in an adult way, or expecting it not to do acts which are part and parcel of infancy. The level of external stress is likely to be high, but the actual fatal assault is always precipitated by some act (however normal or trivial) on the part of the child. This includes crying, refusing food, vomiting, wetting itself, refusing to smile or 'getting in the way'.

There is obviously an overlap between cases of parents causing the death of their child and those in whom violence to the child falls short of a lethal outcome.

Baby battering

This emotive term was coined by Kempe [3] in 1961 as a deliberate effort to arouse public concern. Since then a good deal of research has been done, yet many of the conclusions arrived at by different workers remain contradictory. The incidence of this form of violent crime remains uncertain. A Parliamentary Select Committee appointed to study 'Violence in the Family' reported in 1977 that, in their view, more than 300 children die every year in England and Wales and some 3,000 are seriously injured, with a further 40,000 children suffering mild to moderate injuries. They further estimated that of the seriously injured, some 400 receive injuries which result in chronic brain damage.

The numbers of children at risk must be very great and detection and management of these children and their parents is a major challenge to preventive medicine. One of the greatest problems has been the conflicting attitudes and responses of the various professionals who have become involved in these cases. In many areas special liaison committees have been established to co-ordinate the work of the different social agencies involved and to evolve a coherent response to the problem.

The offenders

While baby battering is not the exclusive perquisite of any single personality profile, or relationship constellation, most studies show almost 90% of parents have many of the following characteristics:

(1)   A history of violence and/or neglect in their own childhood.
(2)   They have broken away from the parental home at an early age.
(3)   They tend to have their first child earlier than the population in general.
(4)   In about a third of cases, the child is illegitimate.
(5)   They tend to select a mate of similar background and similar personality.
(6)   They are socially isolated.
(7)   They have violent outbursts of temper.
(8)   They have unrealistic expectations regarding the child's behaviour.
(9)   They have a history of mental illnesses such as depression or anxiety states.

The more of these factors which are present, the higher the risk to the child.

About 10% of those parents who abuse their children fall into one of the following four sub-groups:

(a) Psychotic parents suffering from some form of delusional illness in which the child is incorporated.

(b) Parents who, though not showing other evidence of a psychosis, hold extreme beliefs in regard to child rearing, perhaps in a pseudo-religious setting.

(c) Cold, affectionless, sadistic psychopaths who self-righteously impose an impossible discipline on their children, punishing them severely for the slightest infractions.

(d) Explosive violent psychopaths who have so little self control that the most minor frustration results in violence totally disproportionate to the circumstances.

Parents who fall into any of these sub-groups cannot safely be left in charge of their children. Treatment is unlikely to be successful in any event and the risk to the child is too high.

Other factors affecting baby battering

Although the vast majority of parents who batter their children have the kind of personality and social characteristics described, the actual offence tends to occur at times of crisis within the family. The other factors which play a part can be considered under the following headings:

1. Social
Battering parents are not more socially disadvantaged than comparable parents who do not batter, and merely relieving their social conditions does not lead to cessation of their offences [4]. However, they seem less able to cope with the problems of child rearing when these are complicated by worries concerning homelessness, overcrowding, poor living conditions, debt and unemployment. Changes for the worse in any of these circumstances can act as the trigger for battering to occur.

2. The child
A child born to reluctant parents at an inauspicious time is part way to being rejected. Should it also fail to meet the expectations of its parents by being of the wrong sex, or having some undesirable physical

characteristics, the degree of rejection may be greater. Babies who are born after difficult labours, or prematurely, and those who for some reason have to be kept away from the mother in the days following delivery, seem to have a greater risk of rejection.

The rejecting mother may in turn handle the child in such a way that she inhibits those activities which normally help to form a bond between mother and child and produces in the child responses which the mother in turn sees as being rejection.

One of the two major factors in child behaviour which seem to lead to breaking point on the parents, part are crying and soiling.

The mother may regard crying by the child as being a deliberate criticism of her. The father may also be very intolerant of crying and demand that the mother stop the child from doing so. She, in turn, becomes over-anxious, the child responds to her tensions, and cries all the more. Crying may also be made more of a problem if it disturbs the neighbours who in turn complain to the mother. As so often the crying takes place at night, the parents' resistance to stress is lowered by the resultant fatigue. Advice from the doctor or health visitor under these circumstances 'to let him cry, he'll settle after a few nights' can be disastrous.

3. The crisis
The actual violence to the child may be part of a continuing regular 'disciplining' but in many cases it is an explosive event that occurs at a time of particular stress within the family. The stress may be social or it may arise as a result of some row between the parents. The mother having tried to cope all day may tell the father that it is his responsibility to stop the child crying—and he in turn responds with the only technique he knows, which is to use his superior strength.

Spouses in child battering families tend to have little capacity for mutual support, and the child becomes the outlet for the anger which each parent may be unable to express toward the other.

Generally where both parents are involved in caring for the child one is the active abuser, while the other encourages, condones, or ignores the abuse.

4. Lack of help
While in theory there may be many agencies available to help them the parents seem to have difficulty in using these effectively. In part this is due to the parents' own difficulty in trusting people, or their own lack of verbal skills. In a surprising number of cases, however, one or other

parent has drawn the attention of a social agency to the problem, even in an indirect way. The failure lies with the professional, who for a number of reasons may ignore the evidence presented. This fact has emerged in the enquiries that have been held as a consequence of some disaster in which the child has died.

One of the most difficult decisions in cases of child abuse is whether or not to separate the children from their parents, and if so, for how long. Such decisions should be made only after the fullest discussion with all the professionals involved and the parents themselves. The child may be kept in a place of safety in the short term to allow time for proper assessment of the parents and the social factors involved.

Kempe [5] has drawn up a check list which may help in arriving at a decision. The more positive answers there are to the questions the greater the risk of repeated abuse and the greater the danger to the child.

(1) Was the parent repeatedly beaten or deprived as a child?
(2) Does the parent have a history of mental illness or criminal activity?
(3) Has the parent been suspected of child abuse in the past?
(4) Is the parent suffering from loss of self esteem, social isolation or depression?
(5) Is the parent experiencing multiple stress (recent divorce, marital discord, financial problems, housing difficulties, etc. etc.)?
(6) Does the parent have a violent temper?
(7) Does the parent have rigid unrealistic expectations of the child?
(8) Does the parent punish the child harshly?
(9) Does the parent see the child as difficult or provocative?
(10) Does the parent reject the child?
(11) Is the parent on drugs or using alcohol?

There is a tendency for professionals to want to think well of their clients in spite of evidence to the contrary. There is also a persistent belief in the myth that blood parents are *always* the best people to care for their children.

In cases of child abuse, the first responsibility must be to ensure that no further harm can come to the child. In the words of Polansky [6], 'this is an area in which social, medical and legal action must be authoritative, intrusive and insistent'.

Wife battering

Until the Matrimonial Causes Act of 1878, husbands had almost a free hand in how they treated their wives. Prior to that Act they were entitled forcibly to return them to the home if they deserted and could physically restrain them from further attempts at escape. The Act gave magistrates the power to order a judicial separation with maintenance and custody of the children to wives whose husbands had seriously assaulted them.

In practical terms, however, it was often extremely difficult for a wife to leave her battering husband.

In 1975 after a sustained campaign led by Mrs Erin Pizzey, a Select Committee was set up to look into the question of violence in marriage. The Committee soon found that there was very little information available to it on this topic.

In 1974, Faulk [7] published a report on 23 men who were remanded in custody for serious assaults on their wives. Eight were charged with murder but at trial this was reduced to manslaughter. The group could be divided into those over the age of 40 and those under this age. The over 40s almost all showed evidence of serious psychiatric disorder, while in the younger age group about half had a psychiatric disturbance and most of these were personality or neurotic disorders. This group obviously represents the extreme end of the spectrum of 'battering husbands' and the findings may not apply to those who keep their violence within some kind of limit. Faulk categorised these men into five groups:

(1) *Dependent, passive*
This type of man tried hard to please a demanding and querulous wife. The violence was explosive and followed a specific act by the victim.

(2) *Dependent, suspicious*
This group were similar to the morbidly jealous described under this heading in connection with murder, though in some cases the jealousy did not have the full delusional intensity but was pervading the relationship.

(3) *Violent and bullying*
These men used violence and threats to gain their ends in most aspects of their lives. This group also showed evidence of alcoholic problems.

(4) *Dominating husbands*
Often successful in other aspects of their lives, these men seemed to regard their wives as subordinates who must obey orders without question. Then violence might be precipitated by trivial events which they regarded as a threat to their authority.

(5) *Normally stable and affectionate husbands*
In this group the violence occurred only at times of mental illness, characteristically during a depressive episode.

Research into battering husbands is obviously very difficult. Few are prepared to co-operate except when in custody, and these are an unrepresentative sample. Evidence tends to be based on statements from battered wives, which while generally accurate, may underplay the wives' own contribution.

Gayford [8] in 1957 reported a series of 100 battered wives. He defined a battered wife as 'a woman who has received deliberate, severe and repeated demonstrable physical injury from her marital partner'.

In 44% of his cases, the offences occurred regularly when the man was under the influence of alcohol. The wounds were usually inflicted with the fists or by kicking, but in 20% attempts had been made at manual strangulation. Almost half claimed that on occasions some form of weapon had been used.

A quarter of the women had been battered by their partner before they began co-habiting. Eighty-five per cent had sexual intercourse prior to marriage and 60% were pregnant when the relationship became more permanent.

Almost half described their own childhood as happy, but this must be viewed with some doubt. Only 65% were brought up by their own parents to the age of 15. In 23% violence had been a feature of their parents' relationship. Seventy per cent of the wives had been treated by their GP's for symptoms of depression or anxiety. Forty-two per cent had made suicide attempts. Few had revealed to the doctor their husband's violence.

Well over half regarded their husbands as jealous men on the basis that they accused the wife of having affairs, checked her activities, claimed she flirted or accused her of being pregnant by other men. While the wives denied the truth of these accusations, 17% admitted to having other sexual relationships while cohabiting with the battering partner.

Effect on children of inter-parent violence

An NSPCC study [9] suggested that at least 80% of the children in such families were adversely affected by the violence. A further factor in their disturbance was the frequent moves from place to place which resulted from rows and fights.

Many of the children had school problems, some being violent and anti-social. Some had psychosomatic symptoms, some get 'accidentally' injured by getting in the way when conflict rages.

Infanticide

A mother who kills her child may be charged with murder, manslaughter, or, under special circumstances, 'infanticide'.

The Infanticide Act 1938 Section 1 (1) states:

> 'Where a woman by any wilful act or omission causes the death of her child being a child under the age of twelve months, but at the time of the act or omission the balance of her mind was disturbed by reason of her not having fully recovered from the effect of giving birth to the child or by reason of the effect of lactation consequent upon the birth of the child, then, notwithstanding that the circumstances were such that but for this Act the offence would have amounted to murder, she shall be guilty of an offence, to wit of infanticide, and may for such offence be dealt with and punished as if she had been guilty of the offence of manslaughter of the child.'

This Act was an amendment of the 1922 Infanticide Act, which limited this defence to the killing of 'a newly born' child, without defining the time limits of 'newly born'.

The Act is a rather curious piece of legislation in a number of ways. First it singles out a specific criminal act to make an assumption that the perpetrator is in an abnormal state of mind. It then removes this mental state as a ground for acquittal, or for a verdict of 'guilty but insane' and substitutes a lesser crime for which she may be punished.

Unlike a murderer who pleads insanity or diminished responsibility, the mother who commits infanticide does not have to show that her act arose as a consequence of her mental state, but only that at the time her mental state was disturbed as a result of the birth or subsequent lactation.

Another curious feature of the act is that a woman who kills two or more of her children during the twelve months following the birth of one of them may be charged with infanticide in respect of the youngest and manslaughter of the other(s).

The 1938 Act with all its anomalies and imperfections was the culmination of many attempts to bring the law into line with practice. Executions of mothers for the murder of their own babies became extremely rare in the nineteenth century (the last being in 1849). By 1864 it was the regular practice of the Home Office to advise that the death penalty be commuted when the woman convicted had killed her own child while it was less than a year old.

Not all mothers who kill their own children before the age of twelve months are 'mentally unbalanced' at the time, while some mothers who kill their new child later than twelve months after birth are still suffering from some form of psychosis following child birth. From the psychiatric point of view, it is more helpful to divide child murders by mothers on the basis of the apparent motive. Resnick [10] suggested the following classifications:

(1) Unwanted child murder—the child was not desired or is no longer wanted.
(2) Acutely psychotic murder—resulting from hallucination, confusional states, etc.
(3) 'Altruistic' murder—to spare the victim real or imagined suffering.
(4) 'Accidental' murder—arising as part of battered child syndrome.
(5) Spouse revenge murder—a way of making the spouse suffer.

When analysed in this way cases of child murder by mothers fall into two broad groups, those in which the killing occurs on the day of the child's birth and those where the child is more than 24 hours old. Resnick proposed the term neonaticide for the first group. In his study he found that about 80% of neonaticides were committed because the child was unwanted, while about 10% were committed by acutely psychotic mothers. In murders of children over 24 hours old, however, over half were committed for 'altruistic' reasons, and a quarter while the mother was acutely a psychotic. The majority of women committing 'altruistic' killings were suffering from depressive disorders and about a third of them accompanied the killing with a suicide attempt. It is only those cases in which, irrespective of whether the child is more than 24 hours old, there is evidence of mental disturbance which fall into the legal category of infanticide.

Unwanted child murder

Mothers who kill their child because it is unwanted, tend to do so during the first 24 hours of its life, often immediately following delivery. Popular methods of killing are strangulation and drowning, the latter being accomplished by placing the baby head down in a toilet—although drowning in milk has also been tried. Mothers in this group tend to be younger than other filicides (more being under 25) and the vast majority are unmarried. The problems associated with having an illegitimate baby are still the primary reason for neonaticide.

There seem to be two sub-groups in the neonaticides. The largest group comprises women who are immature and passive. They become pregnant through failure to take any contraceptive precautions and once pregnant tend to deny the reality of their situation, not seeking abortions, nor making any preparations for the arrival of the child. Some of these mothers are of limited intelligence. The second sub-group tend to be much more forceful women with high sexual drive and resulting promiscuity. They are callous and self-centred and their crime is premeditated and often planned with skill and care.

'Altruistic' filicide

A small number of children are killed by their mothers to spare them *real* suffering (usually referred to as 'mercy killings'). Such mothers show no evidence of any psychiatric disorder and may have reached their decision after long and careful consideration. The vast majority of 'altruistic' killings are done as a result of delusional beliefs held by one or both parents. Most commonly their delusions form part of a depressive illness. To spare the child, the sufferer decides that her only course is to kill herself, and feels that it is not right to leave the child behind. Other depressives suffer from the delusional belief that they and their family are bound to suffer some dreadful fate and that it is kinder to kill the children to spare them from this calamity.

A small number of mothers suffering from paranoid disorders kill their children to prevent them being harmed by an imaginary persecutor.

Acutely psychotic filicide

This group overlaps with the deluded altruistic killers, but the crime tends to be much more impulsive, and either motiveless or based on bizarre motives. It includes cases of schizophrenia in which the killing is the result of hallucinatory instructions, cases of acute delirium, and epileptic automatism.

'Accidental' filicide

There are cases in which repeated violence is used against the child, but where the death of the child was not the primary aim of the violence. These cases are discussed under 'battered baby syndrome'.

Spouse revenge murder

Such cases are relatively rare. They usually arise as a result of the spouse leaving for another partner and the child becomes the focus for the deserted spouse's rage.

Management of infanticide

The attitude of the Courts to infanticide can be seen from table 6.1 which shows the disposal of cases over the years. Nine out of ten women are either committed to hospital or put on probation, often with a condition of psychiatric treatment.

Table 6.1 Disposal of women found guilty of infanticide

	Discharged or bound over	Probation	Imprisonment	Hospital Order etc.
1946–50	24.0%	49.0%	22.7%	4.3%
1951–55	15.0%	55.0%	16.2%	13.8%
1956–60	9.5%	76.2%	3.2%	11.1%
1961–65	5.6%	68.1%	1.3%	25.0%

After Walker and McCabe, *Crime and Insanity in England*, 1973, by courtesy of Edinburgh University Press

'Granny bashing'

It is difficult to estimate how many old people are the victims of deliberate injury inflicted by relatives or other people entrusted with their care. Old people tend to bruise easily and ordinary gripping of their arms when helping them to stand or walk can produce bruising. A push or a slap can give rise to much more serious injury in an old person than a similar assault on a younger person. Violence towards aged relatives is said [12] to be more common in certain situations:

(1) In families where care has been given for long periods of time and where increasing disability finally produces too much stress on the caring relative.
(2) In families where considerable reluctance to take in the old person has been overruled by pressure from outside sources.
(3) Where an almost equally aged spouse has to cope more or less alone with a demented partner.

There is great difficulty in assessing the account given by the old person of the incident. Some will deliberately deny any violence and claim that they fell or knocked into something. Others, however, will invent acts of violence as part of a paranoid illness arising either in a setting of depression, dementia or paraphrenia. The old person with severe memory impairment may be quite unable to remember the circumstances and may confabulate to cover the memory loss. The tale told may claim violence when none occurred, or deny such acts when in reality they took place.

The statement that violence occurred must not be ignored but must be judged in relation to the patient's mental state and other corroboratory evidence. It has been truly said that just because you are paranoid, it does not mean you are NOT being persecuted.

References

Violence within the family

Child battering
1 Scott, P D (1973) *Medicine, Science and the Law*, **13,** 120
2 Scott, P D (1973) Fatal battered baby cases. *Medicine, Science and the Law*, **13,** 197
3 Kempe, C H (1962) *Journal of the American Medical Association*, **181,** 17
4 Smith, S M, Hanson, R and Noble, S (1974) Social aspects of the battered baby syndrome. *British Journal of Psychiatry*, **125,** 568–582
5 Kempe, C H and Kempe, R S (1978) *Child Abuse*. Fontana Books, London

6 Polansky, N and Polansky, N (1968) *Report to the Joint Commission on Mental Health for Children*

Further reading

Kempe, C H (1974) *Helping the Battered Child and his Family*. Lippincott, Philadelphia

Scott, P D (1977) Non-accidental injury in children. *British Journal of Psychiatry*, **131**, 366–380

Carter, J (Ed) (1974) *The Maltreated Child*. Priory Press, London

Helfer, R E and Kempe, C H (1974) *The Battered Child*, 2nd edition. University of Chicago Press

Renvoize, J (1978) *Web of Violence*. Routledge & Kegan Paul, London

Smith, S M and Harrison, R (1975) Interpersonal relationships. Child practices in 214 parents of battered children. *British Journal of Psychiatry*, **127**, 513–525

Olwo, J E and Buchanan, A H (1979) Generations of maltreated children and multi-agency care in one kindred. *British Journal of Psychiatry*, **135**, 289–303

Wife battering

7 Faulk, M (1974) *Medicine, Science and the Law*, **14**(3), 180

8 Gayford, J J (1957) Wife battering. *British Medical Journal*, **1**, 194

9 NSPCC (1978) *Web of Violence*, Renvoize, J. page 143. Routledge & Kegan Paul, London.

Further reading

Scott, P D (1974) *British Journal of Psychiatry*, **125**, 433–441

Pizzey, E (1974) *Scream Quietly or the Neighbours Will Hear*. Penguin Books, Harmondsworth, Middlesex

House of Commons (Session 1974–5) (Session 1975–6) *Minutes of Evidence of Select Committee on Violence in Marriage*. HMSO

Infanticide

10 Resnick, P J (1970) *American Journal of Psychiatry*, **126**, 10

11 Walker, N and McCabe, S (1973) *Crime and Insanity in England, vol 2. New Solutions and New Problems*. Edinburgh University Press

Further reading

d'Orban, P T (1979) Women who kill their children. *British Journal of Psychiatry*, **134**, 560–571

Granny bashing

12 Renvoize, J (1978) *Web of Violence*. Chapter 6, page 113. Routledge & Kegan Paul, London

7. Sexual Offences

Introduction

Sexual conduct is an area of behaviour in which there is considerable disagreement regarding the extent to which criminal law should be involved. In different countries, and at different times in the same country, acts may be considered as criminal, civil wrongs, or purely a matter of private morality. It would seem that in the eyes of the law the only approved form of sexual activity is intercourse *per vaginam* (in conditions of strict privacy) between a legally married man and his wife—and even this is hedged about with some restrictions! Obviously, this legal notion of human sexual activity does not closely match reality.

In practice the legal process is usually evoked in order to try to prevent one or more of the following consequences:

(1) The suffering of physical injury by one of the participants.
(2) The exploitation of persons who are incapable, through youth, or mental disorder, of protecting themselves.
(3) Acts that the majority of people regard as 'unnatural'.
(4) Acts that while acceptable in private between consenting adults would cause shock or distress to other people if performed in public.

The offences that fall within one or more of these general prohibitions will obviously vary in accordance with the general sexual mores of the society at a particular time.

The differing public attitude at different times is reflected in the variety of Acts relating to crimes that have a sexual element. In general, at present, in England and Wales the law relating to sexual offences is contained in the Sexual Offences Act 1956 and the Sexual Offences (Amendment) Act 1976. However, other Acts such as the Mental Health Act 1959, the Indecency with Children Act 1960, and the Vagrancy Act 1823 have sections relating to sexual crimes.

The sexual offences will be discussed under the following headings:

(1)   Sexual offences not involving intercourse
(2)   Those offences involving intercourse.

This is obviously an arbitrary grouping and there is some overlap in both the offences and the offenders.

Of all indictable offences recorded by the police only 0.8% are sexual offences. An indictable offence recorded by the police is said to be cleared up if a person is arrested, summoned or cautioned for the offence, if the offence is attributed to a child under the age of 10, if the offence is taken into consideration by the Court in sentencing the offender on another charge or if the offender cannot be prosecuted, e.g. because he is dead.

The 'clear up rate' for sexual offences is about 78%. This reflects the fact that with the exception of rape, the discovery of the offence is closely associated with the discovery of the offender (e.g. incest)

About half those who are charged with sexual offences plead guilty. Of those who plead not guilty almost 50% are acquitted.

Table 7.1   Sexual Offences 1977

	Offenders found guilty		Cases recorded by police	
	M	F	M	F
Buggery	198	–	594	–
Attempted Buggery	741	–	2,633	–
Indecency between males	1,548	–	1,465	–
Rape	313	–	1,015	–
Indecent assault on females	2,451	11	11,048	
Unlawful sexual intercourse	601	1	3,924	–
Incest	127	2	295	–
Gross indecency with a child	35	3	–	–

Source: *Criminal Statistics England & Wales* (1977) page 34. HMSO.

Offences not involving sexual intercourse

Indecent exposure

The act of exposing the sexual organs in a public place is the subject of two laws, one criminal and one common law.

It is a common law misdemeanour to commit 'an act outraging public decency in public, and in such a way that more than one person sees, or is at least able to see the act'.

Under this law, it is not necessary to prove that more than one person saw the act, but only that two or more people *could* have seen it. It is also not necessary to prove that anyone was actually disgusted or annoyed.

The *mens rea*—the perpetrator need not be shown to have any *sexual* motive, nor any intention to insult in any way. The offence may be committed by a female as well as a male and the exposure need not be to a person of the opposite sex.

Indecent Exposure is also an offence under the 1824 Vagrancy Act:

'. . . every person wilfully, openly, lewdly and obscenely exposing his person with intent to insult any female . . . shall be deemed a rogue and a vagabond'.

Unlike the common law offence, this crime is limited to exposure by a male to a female and requires the specific intent 'to insult'. 'Person' in this context meant 'penis', so however insulting the intent, exposing one's backside did not fall within the provisions of this section. However, this has now changed.

Indecent exposure is one of the commonest sexual offences in England and Wales. The percentage of offences that actually come to Court, however, is very low. Over recent years the number of convictions for indecent exposure has steadily increased. This is unrelated to any change in the law, and at a time when public tolerance of sexual activities has generally increased. For a brief period it seemed as if one form of indecent exposure was about to become the new national sport. 'Streaking' by naked young men (and women) at public events such as cricket matches and the like became an accepted part of the entertainment.

Indecent exposure has usually been regarded as a rather trivial affair, being more of a nuisance than a serious threat. In a percentage of cases, however, the 'exposing' has been a prelude to more serious sexual assaults. The vast majority of 'exposers' do not go on to indulge in other sexual or non-sexual crimes. However, a study of offenders convicted of rape, arson, or robbery with murder (Petri (1969) [1]) showed that 12% had previous convictions for indecent exposure. There was some correlation between the form of exposing and the later more serious crimes. Those cases in which the exposer masturbated at the time and shouted at, or spoke to the victim, or where the victim was also touched or handled in some way had a higher correlation with future violence, than those where only exposure, or exposure with masturbation occurred.

Indecent exposure is the legal term for that form of behaviour which in psychiatric texts is usually referred to as exhibitionism. This term was first used in 1877 by Lasegue [2] in a paper describing seven such cases.

While 'indecent exposers' refers to all those convicted of indecent exposure, exhibitionism is probably better restricted to those who derive sexual satisfaction from the act of exposing their genitals to females without any intention of proceeding to some other sexual act.

Such exhibitionists probably account for the majority of exposers (80% according to Radzinowicz) [3]. The remainder comprise those in whom the exposing is a prelude to other sexual activity, and those very few in whom the exposing is a symptom of a psychotic illness or subnormality of intelligence.

There have been numerous attempts to classify exhibitionists into various categories. Two broad types have been described:

Type 1
Young men of relatively normal personality and good character, who feel impelled to expose themselves in spite of their efforts to control the desire. They tend to feel anxious, guilty and humiliated by their behaviour. They tend to expose a flaccid penis, do not masturbate at the time, and derive little pleasure from the act.

Type 2
Men with more psychopathic traits who derive considerable pleasure from exposing the erect penis, accompanied by masturbation. There is often a sadistic element in their exhibitionism.

Apart from these two main types, and those psychotic or subnormal exposers, there are situational stress exposers. These are men who are normally of good character, free from psychiatric illness, and who under ordinary circumstances had normal adult sexual relationships. Their exposing occurs at times of considerable personal stress, or at times when their normal sexual outlet is denied them. This denial is often due to illness of their wife or other acceptable reasons such as pregnancy. It would seem that they feel too guilty to seek sexual relations with another woman and yet cannot sublimate their sexual drive. Such men often have teenage daughters acting as surrogate 'mother' at the time of their offence, and it is possible that they 'expose' as a way of avoiding incestuous activity. There is some support for this idea in that they not infrequently expose in such a way as to almost guarantee arrest, for example exposing to people who know them, or from their own car on repeated occasions.

Indecent exposure seems to be largely a self limiting condition in that 80% of exposers are only convicted once. However, those who are convicted a second time have a high risk of becoming recidivists.

Additional factors of bad prognostic significance are previous convictions for non-sexual crimes and a predilection for exposing to children.

Indecent assault and indecency with children

In everyday use the term assault is used to cover situations in which the victim either suffers unlawful personal violence, or is led to believe that such violence is about to happen. Strictly, actual violence is the separate crime of battery, as discussed under Offences against the Person, but in indecent assault both threatened and actual violence are included. In order for the assault to be 'indecent' as distinct from a common assault, it must be accompanied by circumstances of indecency on the part of the offender. This indecency may involve the area of the body touched, or it may involve other acts by the perpetrator, including indecent language.

The offence of indecent assault is defined under Sections 14 and 15 of the Sexual Offences Act 1956. It makes it an offence for a 'person' to commit an indecent assault and this clearly includes women.

Indecency with children

This is the subject of a special Act—the Indecency with Children Act 1960, which states:

> 'Any person who commits an act of gross indecency with or towards a child under the age of fourteen, or who incites a child under that age to such an act with him or another, shall be liable on conviction or indictment to imprisonment for a term not exceeding two years or on summary conviction to imprisonment for a term not exceeding six months, to a fine not exceeding one hundred pounds, or both'.

Thus in the case of children under 14, mere incitement is an offence and there is no need for the child to have responded to the invitation.

Indecent assault is a catch all offence which can cover such disparate actions as pinching a passing female's bottom or assault which falls short of rape only because no penile penetration occurred or was attempted.

The cases in which a psychiatrist is asked to see those accused of this offence can be divided into cases of:

(1) Adolescent boys indecently assaulting male or female children.
(2) Adolescent boys indecently assaulting adult females.
(3) Adult males/females indecently assaulting other adults.
(4) Men indecently assaulting male or female children.

1. Adolescent boys indecently assaulting male or female children

Behaviour which would strictly amount to indecent assault were it complained about by the victim forms part of the normal sexual experimentation of young people. There are a number of factors which may lead to the prosecution of a particular individual for acts which in no way differ from those of many of his peers. The following may all contribute singly or in combination:

(1) Lack of social skill.
(2) Lack of personal attractiveness.
(3) Lack of judgement.
(4) Excessive aggressiveness.

These factors may be symptomatic of an underlying mental disorder, the commonest being subnormality of intelligence. Schizophrenia can sometimes lead to similar behaviour. Treatment of the underlying disorder may offer the best chance of avoiding repetition of the offence. Training in social skills and helping the individual extend his normal social contacts with females of his own age can be helpful. In a very small number of cases the offender has some physical deformity which he considers prevents him from developing normal sexual relationships and surgical correction of the abnormality may form a vital part of his management. It is of course important to distinguish between those with actual physical deformities and those who have the delusion that they have some repulsive feature.

In the case of boys with subnormality it is almost impossible to arrange in-patient treatment for them. Most units regard them as being too much of a risk while the special hospitals rightly consider that they in no way require the degree of security offered by such establishments.

2. Adolescent boys who indecently assault adult females

There is obviously some overlap between this group of offenders and the former group. However a number of such offenders do not show any evidence of subnormality of intelligence or of psychiatric illness.

They resemble the group described as 'over controlled psychopaths' who are responsible for some sexual killings, but lack their degree of aggressiveness. They often have older than average parents with the mother being the dominant parent. Both parents may have excessively puritanical views on sexual activities and the subject is taboo in the family. These boys have difficulty in relating to their peers and may be teased and bullied at school.

Management is similar to that of the previous group, but it is vital that they either be separated from the family, or that the parents are themselves involved in the treatment programme.

3. Adult males (or females) who indecently assault other adults

The first point of differentiation is whether the offence involves an adult of the same or opposite sex.

> 'It is an offence for a man to commit an act of gross indecency with another man, whether it is in public or in private, or to be a party to the commission of an act of gross indecency with another man, or to procure the commission by a man of an act of gross indecency with another man' (Section 13, Sexual Offences Act 1956.)

This provision was modified by the 1967 Act so that it is not an offence for a man to commit buggery or gross indecency with another man, provided that the parties consent, that they have attained the age of 21 years and that the act was done in private.

This Act specifies however that a man suffering from severe subnormality within the Mental Health Act 1959 cannot in law give consent.

The Act does not legalise homosexual acts punishable under the Naval Discipline Act 1957, the Air Force Act 1955 or the Army Act 1955.

'Gross indecency' has not been defined by statute but is usually taken as meaning masturbation.

Lesbianism is not a criminal offence, unless one of the participants is under the age of 16, in which case an indecent assault is committed.

4. Men indecently assaulting male or female children

Sexual offences against children are committed by men of all ages, from all social classes and of all levels of intelligence. A number of such offenders come from those entrusted with the care of children, such as teachers, choir masters and scout leaders. Not all the victims are naive innocents. Studies by Virkkunen [4] and Ingram [5] showed that in a substantial proportion of cases the children's behaviour was seductive or provocative, though this may have been unintentioned or sub-conscious. Offenders may fall into one of the groups described below:

(1) Adolescents who are socially or sexually inadequate.

(2) Adolescents who have themselves been the victim of assaults.

(3) Middle-aged men who have always had difficulty in forming adult sexual relationships.

(4) Elderly men who as a result of ageing can no longer form adult sexual relationships.

(5) Men of subnormal intelligence who may not realise that their actions are unacceptable.

(6) Psychopaths in whom offences against children form part of a widespread anti-social and immoral pattern of behaviour.

(7) Situational offenders—men who normally enjoy adult sexual relationships, but who for some reason are prevented from doing so.

(8) 'True' paedophiles in whom the sexual drive is directed exclusively towards prepubescent or adolescent children. Such offenders often claim high motives for their actions and cannot see that there is anything wrong with their behaviour.

Offences involving sexual intercourse

Rape

The present law is contained in the Sexual Offences (Amendment) Act 1976. A man commits rape if he has sexual intercourse with a woman who at the time did not consent to it and he knew that she did not consent, or was reckless as to whether or not she consented.

A husband can only be convicted of the rape of his wife if they are legally separated. He can, however, be charged as an accomplice if he incites others to rape his wife.

Boys under the age of 14 years are legally considered to be incapable of coitus and would, therefore, be charged with indecent assault.

The absence of consent is an essential part of the *actus reus* and must be proved by the prosecution. The prosecution do not have to show that there was actual *dissent* but only an absence of assent. Thus a man who had intercourse with a woman while she was asleep was found guilty of rape. Deliberately rendering a woman insensible with drink or drugs and having intercourse with her constitutes rape.

Submission extracted by duress does not constitute consent.

Apparent consent induced by fraud is no consent. The Sexual Offences Act 1956 (Section 1 (2)) states that 'a man who induces a woman to have sexual intercourse with him by impersonating her husband commits rape'.

The mens rea

The *mens rea* of rape is the intention to have sexual intercourse with a woman knowing that she does not consent or being reckless whether she consents or not. If it is proved that the act *occurred* there can be no argument that there was no *intention* to have sexual intercourse.

The actus reus

Sexual intercourse is defined in the Sexual Offences Act as being complete upon proof of penetration only. There is no need to prove 'the emission of seed'.

Penetration is the entry of the penis into the vagina or the anus and the slightest degree is enough—the hymen need not be broken.

On an indictment for rape, it is open to the jury, if rape is not proved, to bring in a verdict of attempted rape.

Rape is a form of behaviour that incorporates both sexual and aggressive aspects. Its spectrum extends from intercourse obtained by deception to the most brutal sexual killings. General statements about rape that fail to allow for these differences are not likely to be helpful when considering an individual offender. Sociological studies seem to throw more light on the beliefs and prejudices of the investigators than on the act of rape. In any human relationships there is some degree of dominance versus submission and this is part of a normal sexual relationship. In rape the degree of dominance/submission acceptable to both the participants has been exceeded. The reasons for this happening lie within the individuals concerned, though the act may become overt because of social conditions prevailing at that time.

Thus rape is traditionally associated with victorious armies and may at that time be committed by men who would not act out their fantasies under any other circumstances. However, men who find the notion of rape abhorrent do not commit rape even under these circumstances. Rape occurring under these kinds of social conditions fit into the anomie theory of Durkheim [6]. Anomie represents a breakdown in the organisation of values normally governing the behaviour of members of a group or society. Not only may these rules break down in times of war or revolution but they may also fail when some members of the society are unable to obtain the normal goals of that society by acting within the rules. Thus socially disadvantaged groups within a society may begin to take by force those things they feel they cannot obtain by legitimate means.

Rape is also more likely to be committed by members of subcultures in which overt violence is an accepted, and indeed esteemed, form of behaviour. This cultural factor may be of particular importance in cases of gang rape.

The 'victimology' of rape has attracted a good deal of attention. This probably initially reflected the widely held masculine belief that most women who get raped have either asked for it, or submitted with only token resistance. Recently the rape victim has become the focus for womens' liberationists, some of whom take the opposite and equally false view that all forms of male/female relationships amount to rape.

Svalastoga [7] reported a series of rape victims in which 54% of the offenders were complete strangers to the victim, 21% were brief, superficial or indirect acquaintances, 14% were long-term acquaintances and 8% were relatives.

Far from being willing victims, Amir's [8] study (1971) showed that a quarter are coerced by the threat of injury, and a further quarter threatened with a weapon, about a third of victims were handled roughly, a quarter were physically beaten, most of these being brutally attacked and a further 12% were choked. With the extensive reporting of vicious rapes, particularly rapes ending in murder, it is hardly surprising that many women when faced with such a situation, submit without too much physical resistance.

The actual sexual intercourse is often only part of the overall act; about 25% of rape victims are forced to carry out other sexual activities, such as cunnilingus and fellatio which they may find extremely humiliating.

Various attempts have been made to classify rapists into groups either on the basis of psychological or behavioural types [9, 10]. No classification is entirely satisfactory, but may help in organising the assessment of a particular offender and may be of some prognostic value.

1. Psychopathic rapist

This type probably accounts for 30–40% of rapists. The rape is often impulsive and is one facet of a general inability to delay gratification or to tolerate frustration. The offender's history is likely to show other forms of criminality, a poor work record, and involvement with drugs or alcoholism. His relationships with others are likely to be superficial and lacking in consideration for their needs and feelings. His relationship to authority figures is likely to be poor. In general, such rapists tend to use threats and minimal violence to obtain submission. In some cases, however, the rape is part of an aggressive assault and reflects the individual's habitual use of violence to obtain his wishes and dominate others. In some young offenders one finds an isolated sexual offence in an otherwise extensive record. It may be that in such cases the offender did not set out to commit rape, but when disinhibited by the effects of alcohol and aroused by the excitement of other criminal activity (e.g. breaking and entering) he became involved in rape as a secondary activity.

2. Sadistic rapist

These men have a deep-rooted hatred of women, usually arising from their early relationship with their mother or another significant female. The essence of their rape is the infliction of humiliation and suffering on the female. The act of intercourse itself may be trivial. They often demand other humiliating acts and may inflict mutilating injuries on their victims. Their rapes are often carefully planned and they take precautions to ensure the possibility of getting away without detection. This group includes some of the rape murderers.

3. The sexually inadequate (Masculine Identity Conflict)

Members of this group may suffer from considerable uncertainty about their masculinity. Some are overt homosexuals, others have marked fears that they are homosexual. They may be timid shy young men lacking in general social skills and particularly poor at making ordinary contacts with women of their own age. Their offence usually comes as a complete surprise to their friends and relatives. The offence itself is not usually impulsive, but has been fantasised in advance. The victim may be selected as being particularly sexually arousing to the offender.

There is a sub-group of sexually inadequate rapists who cover their sexual doubts by a display of excessive masculinity, bragging about their sexual prowess and indulging in narcissistic activities like body building.

This group find forced submission an important part of rape and may use excessive force to achieve it.

4. The stress rapist

A small number of rapists present a history of extreme situational stress during the period immediately preceding the rape. In general, this type of rapist has led a previously normal sexual life and has engaged in no other criminal activities. Following the rape he may express considerable guilt and remorse and may try to make some recompense to his victim. There is often an overlap between this type and the psychopathic rapists, depending on the degree of personality disorder in the offender.

5. The psychotic

This group constitutes less than 10% of all rapists. From the psychiatric point of view they form an important group, both because of the legal implication of their insanity and also because adequate control of the psychotic illness may lead to the cessation of rape activity. The most common psychotic illness associated with rape is probably mania. The rape committed by a psychotic is sometimes bizarre, violent and often extremely terrifying for the victim.

Some rapes end in murder, though fortunately this is relatively rare. It is possible to distinguish two types of sex killing. First there are those rapists who kill for non-sexual reasons, that is they kill to prevent subsequent identification by their victim. They derive no sexual satisfaction from the act of killing and do not perform any sexual acts on their dead victim. Usually they do not mutilate the body. Secondly, there are those for whom the killing is the sexually arousing part of the act. They may or may not have intercourse with the victim dead or alive. They may, however, experience orgasm during the killing or masturbate afterwards. Some compulsively dismember or disembowel their victim. There is a likelihood of repeated offences in these cases, and the characteristics of the lust murder have been described as:

(1) Periodic outbursts due to returning compulsive sexual desires.
(2) Nearly always cutting and stabbing, particularly of the breasts or genitals, frequently with sucking or licking of the wounds, biting of the skin, and sometimes drinking of blood or eating the flesh of the victim.
(3) Often no attempt at intercourse with the victim but evidence of ejaculation.
(4) Normal behaviour between outbursts.

Such crimes obviously pose enormous problems for the police and form the subject of much popular speculation. The crimes sometimes cease without explanation and it is assumed that the perpetrator has committed suicide or been incarcerated in some institution as a result of other crimes or of being found insane.

Revitch [11] reviewed 43 such cases and described the following characteristics:

(1) An hostility to women in general.
(2) A preoccupation with maternal sexual conduct.
(3) Overt or covert incestuous preoccupation.
(4) Guilt over, and rejection of, sex as impure.
(5) Ideas of sexual inferiority.
(6) A need to 'completely possess' the victim or whatever she may represent.

In another study Reinhardt [12] points out that while the sex killer may have committed previous offences these usually do not arouse suspicion that he is likely to kill in the future. He is often regarded as being well mannered, timid, gentle, reserved and religious. The majority seem to be borderline psychotics whose grasp of reality is tenuous and at times breaks down completely in an explosive way.

Sex killing attracts considerable publicity and may give rise to imitative behaviour. This may be the result of a similarly unstable individual being provoked into acting out his own fantasies or it may be an opportunist who, having killed for his own reasons, tries to make it look like the work of the current 'Jack the Ripper' in order to distract attention from himself. Such cases also produce a number of false confessions from mentally disordered persons who may be referred for psychiatric investigation.

Gang rape

In about 30% of cases of rape there is more than one offender involved. In half of these cases there are two aggressors involved and in the remainder there are three or more. Many of the victims of gang rapes are prostitutes, or girls who have associated promiscuously with members of the gang on an individual basis previously. Alcohol intake is a significant factor in both offender and victim of gang rapes.

Incest

Incest was not a common law offence until 1908. Until that date it was dealt with by the Ecclesiastic Courts. The law relating to this offence was updated in the Sexual Offences Act 1956 as follows:

'S.S.10
(1) It is an offence for a man to have sexual intercourse with a woman whom he knows to be his granddaughter, daughter, sister or mother.

(2) In the foregoing sub-section 'sister' includes half-sister, and for the purposes of that sub-section any expression importing a relationship between two people shall be taken to apply notwithstanding that the relationship is not traced through lawful wedlock.

S.S.11

(1) It is an offence for a woman of the age of 16 or over to permit a man whom she knows to be her grandfather, father, brother or son to have sexual intercourse with her by her consent. Brother in this sub-section, having the same qualification as sister in 10 (2)'.

The degree of consent required of the woman to make her a party to incest would seem to be greater than that required to negate a charge of rape. The Courts have distinguished between 'submission' and 'permission' in such cases.

The essential features of the crime are that the individuals concerned must fall within the specified relationships, that at least one of them must be aware of that relationship and that sexual intercourse as previously defined in the Act, must have occurred.

Incest between consenting adults has been regarded as being a matter of private morality and thus not suitable for criminal sanctions. It has also been argued that children are sufficiently protected from incestuous relationships by the laws prohibiting sexual intercourse with minors. At present, however, it is an act of illegal intercourse in its own right.

Prevalence
Incest, particularly father-daughter incest seems to have occurred in all types of civilisations throughout recorded history. In the vast majority of societies there have been strict taboos against the practice, though there have been certain limited exceptions in which such relationships were actively required among the ruling families.

Of all crimes, incest is probably the one in which the official figures for reported offences under-estimate the true prevalence. The majority of known cases are not reported to the police, but come to the notice of doctors, social workers and priests. Even these 'known' cases probably represent a small fraction of cases actually occurring.

There was a gradual increase in the number of cases known to the police between the 1908 Act and the mid-1960s. Since that time the number has remained fairly static at about 300 to 350 cases per year. Only about half of these cases actually come to trial.

The most commonly occurring cases are brother-sister relationships, but few of these come to official attention. The vast majority of cases reported are of father-daughter incest. Mother-son incest does not occur very often either, or is rarely reported in the literature, in spite of its supposed psychoanalytic importance.

The under-reporting of incestuous relationships is in part due to the essentially 'private' nature of the crime, and in part due to the conspiracy to remain silent shared by the perpetrator, the victim, and often other members of the family. Estimates have placed the percentage of reported cases as being as low as 5% of offences committed. With such low 'reportage' rates, it is extremely difficult to be sure about changes in the actual incidence of the crime, as a relatively small change in the percentage reported will appear to represent a large change in the incidence of the offence.

The low reported rates also render any sociological factors difficult to assess. Reported cases contain an over-representation of lower socio-economic groups, but the offence is often discovered while investigating some other suspected crime. Thus it may be that factors related to 'discovery' are being described rather than factors relevant to the act itself.

Social Class and Housing
Incest is not confined to any one social class. The highest incidence of reported incest is found among working class families living in poor housing conditions in towns. Over-crowding has been stated to be a factor in the aetiology of incest by a number of investigators [13]. However, cases certainly occur in families living in perfectly adequate social conditions.

Father-daughter incest

The fathers
Studies of incestuous fathers are limited as the majority of cases come to light in a way which makes assessment of the father difficult. Those studies based on reported cases suffer from the drawback of probably being unrepresentative of the total population of incestuous fathers. Such studies as have been reported do, however, show fairly consistent findings.

Gebhard et al [14] reported that only about 10% of most offenders had IQ's below 70%.

Mental illness *per se* has also been found to be uncommon in incestuous fathers. The majority of such fathers do, however, show many of the features generally regarded as forming the constellation of personality traits labelled psychopathic. There is a separate group of offenders who seem to be relatively normal personalities, in whom the incestuous relationship occurs for a very limited time, for only a few occasions, and when normal sexual relations with their wife has for some reason been impossible.

Psychopathic group
This group can be further sub-divided into aggressive and inadequate psychopaths.

The aggressive incestuous father is likely to be in his 40s and to have a history of alcoholism and previous criminal offences [15]. He is described as violent and irritable by his family and workmates, and generally has a poor work record with frequent job changes and long periods of unemployment [16]. His sex drive is high and the incest offences often involve more than one daughter at a time. The offences occur when normal sexual relationship with the wife is also continuing, and sometimes when a current 'mistress' is also in residence.

The fathers are themselves often from 'broken homes', and have left the nuclear family at an early age. They have generally had little formal education. The first incestuous offence often occurs as a drunken assault on the daughter in the wife's temporary absence.

'Inadequate' psychopathic fathers
In this group the father has a similar history of an unsatisfactory childhood, and a poor work record. The reasons for failure in employment are likely to be due to repeated absences on account of illnesses of dubious physical causation such as 'back-ache', or of neurotic disorders with somatic manifestations. In many instances this ill health will have freed the wife to adopt the role of breadwinner and the husband, to a greater or lesser extent, takes on the housewifely duties. While alcohol plays a part in the occurrence of incestuous acts, these are less likely to involve violence and more likely to involve a trading on the daughter's sympathy for, and duty to, the poor, hard done-by father.

'Normal' fathers
In some 30% of reported cases, the father does not show any evidence of mental illness or psychopathic disorder.

In this group the offences tend to occur for a very limited time and on only a few occasions, usually at a time when for some reason a normal sexual relationship with the wife is impossible. Differentiation of this group from the psychopathic group is prognostically important.

Predisposing factors which may contribute to the development of an incestuous relationship include:

(1) Any situation in which an adolescent daughter takes on the role of surrogate mother following the loss of the real mother through death, divorce, or separation.

(2) Social isolation due to geographic factors, poverty or cultural differences.

(3) Marital disharmony, or the breakdown of ordinary marital sexual relations.

(4) Alcoholism.

(5) Gross overcrowding leading to loss of privacy and inadvertent sexual contact.

Wives of incestuous men

In many cases the wife is aware of the incest between her husband and daughter [17] and in some instances gives it tacit encouragement. In other instances, while not giving tacit encouragement, the wife creates a situation in which incest is more likely to occur by denying her husband sexual activity and at the same time encouraging her elder daughter to play an increasingly 'maternal' role in the family. Others have evening or night jobs, which leave husband and daughter alone at home overnight. This is sometimes found in cases where the wife has known of previous incestuous events with a daughter who has subsequently left home.

In spite of what has been said above, it is important to remember that in perhaps 30% of cases the personality of both parents seems to be quite normal. The claims of the 'victim' should not be regarded as unfounded merely because the father does not conform to the expected personality profile.

The daughters

It is extremely difficult to predict the effect an incestuous relationship will have on the girl. The outcome may be greatly modified by her basic personality, the circumstances of the relationship, other people's attitudes, and her own subsequent experiences.

Psychotic illness arising from incestuous relationships seems to be rare. A number of girls seem to develop personality disorders themselves, but this may be due to inherited factors and/or the generally disturbed upbringing they had of which the incest formed only a part.

Some girls develop an aversion to sexual activity which may create problems within their marriages or may lead them to avoid marriage altogether. Other girls, however, appear to become promiscuous and sometimes seem to seek substitutes for the incestuous relationship by pursuing older men.

Yet others appear to suffer no lasting ill effects and establish perfectly satisfactory sexual relationships and lead totally normal lives.

The proportion of 'victims' who fall into the above groups varies between different studies.

Brother/Sister incest

Such cases are rarely reported but every psychiatrist sees a number of female patients who 'confess' to having had sexual intercourse with a brother at some time during puberty. The youngest daughter in a large family of brothers would seem to be the most vulnerable. The incidence is highest in families where there is lack of paternal control and supervision, often due to the physical absence of the father.

Mother/Son incest

In spite of the emphasis on the Oedipal complex in analytic literature, there are very few reported cases of overt sexual intercouse between mother and son. The majority of reported cases show that one or other of the participants was mentally disordered at the time. This may reflect the fact that where both parties are mentally normal, the boy does not complain and thus draw outside attention to the offence.

Genetic aspects

Breeding between closely related individuals increases the chance of the off-spring inheriting recessive genes which may produce some congenital abnormality. The risk to the child is difficult to quantify because the majority of children born as a result of incest will not be recognised as such. Studies of cases of known incestuous pregnancies are rather alarming.

The mothers are themselves generally very young, which of itself increases the risk of mortality and morbidity in the child. Adams [18] reported a study which showed in 18 incestuous births, 5 were stillborn or died in early infancy, 2 were severely retarded and 3 were of borderline I.Q. Carter (1967) [19] reported on 13 children and found that 8 had serious congenital abnormalities, 3 of whom had died.

Management of suspected cases of father-daughter incest

Social Services Departments have a statutory duty to inform the police of suspected cases of incest under the Children's and Young Persons Act 1969. The Social Services Department may remove the child into care if it is thought that the child is in moral danger. When the police are involved and the father charged, he is either remanded in custody or allowed bail on condition that he stays away from his wife and child for the duration of the bail. Remanded in custody is relatively rare. The majority of fathers so charged plead guilty.

Of cases reported to the police about half actually come to court, and a good deal of discretion is used in deciding on prosecution. In those cases where prosecution leads to conviction, the majority receive a prison sentence of 1 to 3 years—a smaller number receive sentences of 5 to 7 years. These longer sentences tend to be given where the incest involves younger children.

Hospital orders are very rarely made, but suspended sentences and probation are now being more frequently used.

It has been suggested that the effects of the trial, sentence and break-up of the family may have more adverse effect on the child than the incestuous relationship itself.

In parental incest there is obviously some overlap between offenders who also have sexual relationships with children to whom they are not related in such a way as to bring it within the orbit of incest. Also there is an overlap with parents who, while not having actual intercourse with their children, indulge in other activities which are also proscribed by law. These crimes are discussed later.

The major difference between sexual acts within the nuclear family and those involving 'outsiders' is that in the former case the dynamics involve the whole family, while in the latter it is the psychodynamics of the offender which are of major importance. Case work with the family has been claimed to have some degree of long-term success.

Sexual offences involving children

It is obvious that there are a group of offenders whose crimes involve children. They may commit offences which range from indecent exposure, or indecency, through indecent assault, to actual sexual intercourse (either as an incestuous relationship or with non-relatives with the connivance of the victim) or as rape and rape murder. While there is a continuum of offences from the relatively trivial to the most horrific, the majority of offenders do not progress from one act to the next, but remain more or less consistent in their transgressions. However, a small minority who start with indecent exposure end up committing sexual killings. In attempting to assess the dangerousness of a sexual offender, factors other than the nature of the sexual crime must be taken into account.

There has in the past been a tendency to assume that the majority of child sexual abuse was perpetrated by men who had an exclusive preference for pre-pubertal children as a source of sexual gratification. Such men being labelled paedophiles.

In discussing the assessment of the individual who is charged with a sexual offence against children, it is convenient to consider the totality of offenders, and then to consider the special features of specific offences.

One of the primary questions that the Court will wish to ask is, 'what is the likelihood of the offence being repeated?'. In order to attempt an answer to this question, two main factors must be assessed. First, to what extent does the offence arise from internal psychological factors as compared to external environmental factors? Second, what environmental factors were relevant to the offence and what is the chance of these factors recurring? To arrive at answers to these questions consideration must be directed to a number of issues which are discussed below:

1. The length of history of the behaviour
It is well known that the best guide to a person's behaviour in the future is his behaviour in the past. Thus the longer and more frequent the offender's sexual activities have involved children, the more likely he is to continue in the same way.

2. The basic sexual orientation of the offender
Where the history reveals exclusively paedophilic sexual activities, the likelihood of repetition is higher than in cases where it represents a regression from adult (to adult) sexual relationships.

3. What factors may have lead to a change in sexual behaviour?
In cases where the offence represents a regression from adult/adult

sexuality, it is important to explore any factors which may have contributed to the change and to assess the extent to which they continue or will continue to operate. Precipitating factors may be found in all areas of the perpetrator's life situation.

Obviously, changes in the nature or availability of his normal sexual outlet are likely to be of primary importance. The loss by death or separation of his sexual partner is an obvious example, but the less obvious withdrawal of sexual activity by a partner as the result of illness, pregnancy or loss of desire may have to be enquired about. Notions of virility and potency are involved not only in the direct sexual role but also in almost all activities which involve the status of the individual. Thus events which diminish the individual's idea of his own ability in any area may lead to self doubts about his sexual capacity. This in turn may lead him to select a sexual partner whom he can easily dominate and who will not be critical of his actual sexual performance. These attributes may most easily be met by selecting a child as the sexual object.

When the precipitating factor can be identified with reasonable certainty, it is then possible to predict the likelihood of repetition on the basis of whether the precipitating cause continues to operate, or whether it can be substantially modified.

4. Other contributory factors
Many offenders claim that they only act out sexually with children while under the influence of drugs or alcohol. In such cases it is important to try and assess the extent to which they have a drink problem in its own right (see Alcoholism, chapter 15). It is important to try and distinguish between such a person and the offender who takes drink, even excessively, in order to give himself courage to commit the offence, or to deliberately provide himself with an excuse if caught.

5. Degree of access to children
The risk of repetition is obviously higher where the offender has easy, frequent and regular contact with his actual or potential victims. There are few things more difficult to resist than temptation.

6. The offender's emotional attitude to his offence
The less actual emotional distress the offender feels about his offence the more likely he is to offend again. The psychological defences employed may range through total denial, projection of guilt on to the victim, to rationalisation. The less the subjective feeling of guilt and

remorse, the greater the likelihood of repetition. It is important to try and distinguish between expressed remorse and felt remorse.

7. *What effect has the charge had on his life situation?*
Some offenders experience a sense of relief when activity which has been a source of private guilt for them finally emerges into public knowledge. They are keen to use the opportunity for getting help with their problems and readily accept the need for both the punishment and treatment. Some are anxious to adopt the role of a 'sick' individual in order that they may escape the consequences of their actions, and once this has been achieved they promptly deny their need for treatment.

In addition to considering these specific points in trying to assess the likelihood of repetition, it is necessary to consider all the other personality features of the individual which may be relevant, so that an inventory of his strengths and weaknesses can be compiled and a balance struck between the two.

Areas of particular concern are:

(a) *Capacity to exercise self control*
The degree to which the individual can control his aggressive drive is obviously highly important. A history of frequent non-sexual assaults on children or adults, self mutilation or injury, or suicide attempts, all suggest a limited degree of control.

A history of impulsive decisions in respect of work or relationships, or of recklessness in regard to money, alcohol, drugs or driving may also indicate impulsiveness and lack of self discipline, and hence a greater likelihood to reoffend if presented with the opportunity.

(b) *Intolerance of frustration*
In the case of the individual who seems to offend only when subject to some form of stress, it is important to determine what level and what nature of stress seems to exceed his ability to cope. Thus a history of his response to various stresses at different times in his life may be illuminating.

The capacity to exercise self control and to tolerate frustration may be demonstrated by the ability to set and achieve long term goals. Success or failure in this may provide some indication of the offender's relative capacity.

(c) *Psychiatric disorders*
A small percentage of sexual offenders commit their offences while

suffering from a clinically overt psychiatric illness. By the time they present for psychiatric examination, many will be showing evidence of depressive or anxiety reactions to the situation in which they find themselves. It is important to try and distinguish between these cases. An objective history from family doctors, hospital records, accounts of employers may provide some clarification. Histories obtained from interested parties such as parents or spouse must be assessed with an awareness of the informant's emotional involvement.

The disorders most likely to be relevant are manic depressive illness and schizophrenia and the usual symptoms of these conditions must be sought. Organic brain disorders may also present in this way and an assessment of intellectual function should form a standard part of the examination. The possibility of some transient disorder of cerebral activity should always be considered and appropriate investigations initiated in those cases where the history or examination provides some evidence in favour of their presence.

Other offences involving sexual intercourse

The offences include those referred to as 'unnatural' offences, and technical offences. The latter are not usually of special psychiatric interest except that it may be necessary to give evidence as to the victim's mental state or intelligence.

Unnatural offences

Buggery
Buggery is the act of anal intercourse *per anum* by a man with a man or woman; or intercouse *per anum* or *per vaginam* by a man or a woman with an animal. It can be committed by a husband with his wife. As in rape, penetration must be proved, but ejaculation need not. Consent is no defence, in fact the consenting party is also guilty. The person carrying out the intercourse is called the 'agent' and the recipient is the 'patient'.

In the 1956 Sexual Offences Act it was an offence under Section 12 (1) 'for a person to commit buggery with another person or with an animal'.

This was modified by the Sexual Offences (Amendment) Act of 1976 which made it no longer an offence for a man to commit buggery or gross indecency with another man, so long as:

(1) The act is done in private.
(2) The parties consent.
(3) Both parties are over the age of 21 years.

This gives rise to the curious situation that a man cannot legally have anal intercourse with his consenting wife even in private, but may bugger his best friend under similar circumstances.

Special laws apply to homosexual offences between members of the armed forces.

Indecency between men

Section 13 of the Sexual Offences Act 1956 states:

> 'It is an offence for a man to commit an act of gross indecency with another man whether in public or private, or to be a party to the commission by another man of an act of gross indecency with another man, or to procure the commission by a man of an act of gross indecency with another man'.

This has been amended by the 1976 Act to allow such acts between consenting adults in private. The nature of 'gross indecency' and the distinction between it and 'indecency' is not clearly defined. It comprises sexual acts not involving anal intercourse and includes mutual masturbation, oral-genital contact and intercrural contact.

Solicitation by men

Under Section 32 of the Sexual Offences Act 1956

> 'It is an offence for a man persistently to solicit or importune in a public place for immoral purposes'.

The sentence for this offence is considerably harsher than that for the similar crime if committed by women.

(See Homosexuality and Paedophilia in Chapter 18, Sexual Deviation.)

Intercourse with a girl under thirteen

Section 5 of Sexual Offences Act 1956 states:

> 'It is an offence for a man to have unlawful sexual intercourse with a girl under the age of thirteen'.

It is no defence under this Section for the man to believe that the girl was over thirteen, however reasonable such a belief might be.

Intercourse with a girl under sixteen
Section 6 of the 1956 Act makes it an offence to have intercourse with a girl under the age of sixteen even with her consent unless the man believes her to be his legal wife, or if he is under the age of 24, has not been previously charged with a similar offence and has reasonable grounds for believing her to be over sixteen.

Intercourse with a defective
Section 7 of the Sexual Offences Act 1956 as amended by the Mental Health Act of 1959 provides:

'1. It is an offence, subject to the exception mentioned in this Section, for a man to have unlawful sexual intercourse with a woman who is a defective.
2. A man is not guilty of an offence under this Section because he has unlawful sexual intercourse with a woman if he does not know and has no reason to suspect her to be a defective'.

Defective in this section means a person suffering from severe subnormality as defined in the 1959 Mental Health Act:

'a state of arrested or incomplete development of mind which includes subnormality of intelligence and is of such a nature or degree that the patient is incapable of living an independent life or of guarding himself against serious exploitation, or will be so incapable when of an age to do so'.

Sexual intercourse with mentally disordered patients
Under Section 128 of the Mental Health Act 1959 it is an offence for an officer, employee or manager of a hospital or mental nursing home to have sexual intercourse with a woman receiving treatment in the hospital or home, or if the intercourse is on the premises, who is receiving treatment there as an out-patient. Similarly in the case of a man having intercourse with a woman who is a mentally disordered patient subject to his guardianship or in his custody or care.

References

Sexual Offences

Indecent exposure
1 Petri, H (1969) *Nervenarzt*, **40**, 220
2 Lasegue, (1877) *Union Médicale*, **23**, 709
3 Radzinowicz, L (Ed) (1957) *Sexual Offences*. MacMillan, London

Further reading

Rooth, F G (1971) Indecent exposure and exhibitionism. *British Journal of Hospital Medicine*, **5**(3), 521

Indecent assault and indecency with children
4 Virkkunen, M (1975) Victim-precipitated paedophilic offences. *British Journal of Criminology*, **15**, 175–180
5 Ingram, Fr M (1979) The participating victim I. The participating victim II. *British Journal of Sexual Medicine*, Jan 22–6, Feb 24–6

Further reading

Fitch, J H (1962) Men convicted of sexual offences against children. *British Journal of Criminology*, **3**, 18–37
Rosen, I (Ed) (1964) *The Pathology and Treatment of Sexual Deviation*. Oxford University Press
Law, S K (1979) Child molestations. *Medicine, Science and the Law*, **19**, 55–60
West, D J, Roy, C and Nichols, F L (1978) *Understanding Sexual Attacks*. Heinemann, London

Rape
6 Durkheim, E (1951) *Suicide: A Study in Sociology* (Ed 1951) p 241. The Free Press, New York
7 Svalastoga, K (1962) Rape and social structure. *Pacific Sociological Review*, **5**, 48–53
8 Amir, M (1971) *Patterns in Forcible Rape*. Chicago University Press

Classification of rapists
9 Gibbens, T C N, Way, C and Soothill, K L (1977) Behavioural types of rape. *British Journal of Psychiatry*, **130**, 32–42
10 Rada, R (1978) *Clinical Aspects of the Rapist*. Grune & Stratton, New York

11 Revitch, E (1965) Sex, murder, and the potential sex murderer. *Diseases of the Nervous System*, **26**, 640–648
12 Reinhardt, J M (1961) The sex killer. *Police*, **5**, 10–13

Further reading

Soothill, K L, Jack, A and Gibbens, T C N (1976) Rape: a 22-year cohort study. *Medicine, Science and the Law*, **16** (1), 62–69
Bowden, P (1978) Rape. *British Journal of Hospital Medicine*, **20**/3, 286–290
Submission to Mrs Justice Heilbron's Advisory Group on the Law of Rapes (8th July 1976) *Medicine, Science and the Law*, **16** (3), 154
Abel, G G et al (1977) The components of rapists' sexual arousal. *Archives of General Psychiatry*, **34** (8), 895–903
Groth, A N and Birnbaum, H J (1979) *Men Who Rape*. Plenum Press, New York

Incest
13 Lukanowicz, N (1972) *British Journal of Psychiatry*, **120**, 131
14 Gebhard, P H, Gagnon, J H, Pomeroy, W B and Christensen, C U (1965) *Sex Offenders*. Harper Row, New York
15 Virkkunen, M (1974) *Medicine, Science and the Law*, **14**, 124
16 Marsch, H (1973) *Incest*. André Deutsch, London
17 Weiner, I B (1964) *Criminologica*, **4**, 137
18 Adams, M S, Neet, J U (1967) Children of incest. *Paediatrics*, **40**, 55–62
19 Carter, C O (1967) *Lancet*, **i**, 436

Further reading

Browning, D H (1977) Incest; children at risk. *American Journal of Psychiatry*, **134**, 1, 69–72
Burgess, A W, Groth, N. A. et al (1978) *Sexual Assault of Children and Adolescents*. Lexington Books, Lexington, Mass., USA
Cavallin, H (1966) Incestuous fathers: a clinical report. *American Journal of Psychiatry*, **122**, 1132–1138
Weinberg, S R (1955) *Incest Behaviour*. New York Citadel

8. Offences against Property

Theft and related offences

Until 1968 the laws concerning stealing had evolved in a haphazard way over many hundreds of years. From the very simplistic views expressed in Common Law the law had developed to cope with ever more ingenious methods of dishonesty. This resulted in an extremely complicated set of laws which were difficult to administer. In 1968 the Theft Act was passed which made sweeping and fundamental changes; offences were reformulated, avoiding as far as possible terms which could only be understood by lawyers.

The present laws relating to theft and related offences are defined in the Theft Act 1968 Section 1 (1) as follows:

'A person is guilty of theft if he dishonestly appropriates property belonging to another with the intention of permanently depriving the other of it'.

The *mens rea*

The appropriating of property belonging to another must be done both:

(1) Dishonestly (and)
(2) With the intention of permanently depriving the owner of it.

Such an act is not dishonest if it is done by someone who believes:

'that he has in law the right to deprive the other of it, on behalf of himself or of a third person' or 'that he would have the other's consent if the other knew of the appropriation and the circumstances of it'.

There is no statement in the Act that the belief has to be a reasonable one.

Robbery

Section 8 of the 1968 Theft Act states:

1. 'A person is guilty of robbery if he steals, and immediately before or at the time of doing so, and in order to do so, he uses force on any person or puts or seeks to put any person in fear of being then and there subjected to force'.

Burglary

1. 'A person is guilty of burglary if:
   (a) he enters any building or part of a building as a trespasser and with intent to commit any such offences as are mentioned in subsection (2) below, or
   (b) having entered any building or part of a building as a trespasser he steals or attempts to steal anything in the building or that part of it or inflicts or attempts to inflict on any person therein any grievous bodily harm.
2. The offences referred to in Subsection (1)(a) above are offences of stealing anything in the building or part of the building in question, inflicting on any person therein any grievous bodily harm or raping any woman therein and of doing unlawful damage to the building or anything therein'.

Aggravated burglary

1. 'A person is guilty of aggravated burglary if he commits any burglary and at the time has with him any firearm, imitation firearm, any weapon of offence or any explosive . . .'

Theft

Theft and its related crimes have been one of the few growth industries in post-war Britain as can be seen from Table 8.1.

What the figures do not show is the enormous cost to the country of this criminal activity. A cost to be counted not only in financial terms but also in terms of human suffering for many of the victims. The trauma of finding one's home burgled, or the terror of being robbed by violent criminals can leave a permanent psychiatric scar on the victim as real as any physical injury sustained. The vast majority of such crimes are committed by people with no recognisable form of psychiatric disorder.

Table 8.1 Indictable offences recorded by the police

England and Wales: Number of offences (thousands)

Offence	1969	1970	1971	1972	1973	1974	1975	1976	1977
Burglary	420.8	431.4	451.5	438.7	393.2	483.8	521.9	515.5	604.1
Robbery	6.0	6.3	7.5	8.9	7.3	8.7	11.3	11.6	13.7
Theft and handling stolen goods	911.5	952.6	1003.7	1009.5	998.9	1189.9	1267.2	1285.7	1487.5

Source: *Criminal Statistics, England & Wales* (1977) HMSO

Shoplifting

The form of theft which has roused most interest in psychiatrists seems to be that of 'shoplifting'. This is frequently referred to as if it were a specific crime and it has been suggested that by using this title the activity has been given an aura of respectability that plain 'thieving' lacks. The growth of this crime can be seen from the figures in Table 8.2, and the cost to the community is enormous. There have been many speculations as to the reasons for this increase, but there can be little doubt that the vast majority of shoplifters are motivated by nothing more complicated than greed. Table 8.2 shows how the number of recorded offences of shoplifting more than doubled between 1969 and 1977.

Table 8.2 Shoplifting—Offences recorded (totals)

1969	1970	1971	1972	1973	1974	1975	1976	1977
91,169	101,822	119,281	126,844	130,161	164,063	175,552	180,993	213,276

Source: *Criminal Statistics, England & Wales* (1977) HMSO

Gibbens et al (1971) [1] published a ten-year follow-up study of 886 shoplifters. These were mostly convicted in Central London where the population of shoppers is very different from less cosmopolitan centres. They found that almost a third of the female offenders were young foreigners and that these represented 46% of offenders aged between 17 and 30. The peak age among British women was 51 to 60. Eighty per cent of the women were first offenders whose reconviction rate was 11%.

They found that the admission rate to mental hospitals for middle-aged women convicted of shoplifting was more than three times that of the corresponding population. This reflects the association between shoplifting in the middle-aged with depression. They suggested 'a typical picture of mixed physical and mental symptoms in a woman of 50 who had recently had a hysterectomy and had not felt well since. She has backache, headaches, dizziness, insomnia and a persistent sense of depression. She sometimes gets up in the night to turn off the gas or to see that the door is locked. She has no serious financial difficulties, but her husband and children take no notice of her and she feels that life in the future stretches out like a desert. She has been seeing her doctor regularly and is receiving tranquillisers, but she has not been to see him for three months because she feels she is wasting his time'.

Gibbens estimated that such women accounted for between 10% and 20% of those arrested for shoplifting and that they are convicted only once.

While there can be no doubt that such middle-aged female depressives do account for some cases of shoplifting, they do not exhaust the psychiatric aspects of the crime. Shoplifting does differ in some respects from most other forms of theft. First, it is essentially a very public crime and often occurs in a setting that openly invites the participant to help herself (though there is an expectation that cash will be given in return). Supermarkets and similar establishments deliberately set out to encourage the shopper to take a wide range of articles that may or may not be really needed.

In addition to being large and crowded, such stores often assault the shopper with a battery of powerful stimuli both visual and auditory. Such distracting stimuli may cause inadvertent shoplifting by honest individuals at times when their level of concentration is impaired. This may be due to a lowered awareness or to an increased distractability. Such conditions may be induced by a wide range of physical and mental disorders.

1. Physical illness
People with mild confusional states resulting from extracerebral organic disorders such as infections, or from intracerebral causes such as cerebral atherosclerosis may unintentionally put items of shopping into their own bags rather than the receptacle provided by the store. Sometimes the articles taken may be a rather bizarre collection of items that are not needed or wanted by the person taking them. It is not wise to place too much reliance on this fact in deciding that the 'theft' was

unintentional. Though the offender may be a life long teetotaller, it does not follow that his friends may not enjoy the bottle of whisky hidden in his shopping bag!

2. Other physical illnesses

Though the illness itself may not produce a confusional state, it is possible that drugs taken for its treatment may do so. The list of possible drugs is long but some of the more obvious examples are psychotropic drugs, antihistamines, hypnotics and analgesics. Combinations of drugs may also cause problems, and it is important in all cases to enquire carefully into any medicines taken including those the offender may have purchased without reference to his family doctor.

Anxiety states. Considering how many women claim they feel anxious in supermarkets, it is remarkable that such shops flourish as they do. However, some women do become panic stricken in such environments and become overwhelmed with the need to leave the store as rapidly as possible. Generally, they abandon their loaded basket or trolley, but some charge out clutching unpaid for goods.

Depression and hypomania. In both depressed and hypomanic people the ability to concentrate may be impaired. The depressive preoccupied by worries and sunk in gloom may wander out of a store without paying. The hypomanic distracted by trivial stimuli, overactive and distractable may do the same. Both may also shoplift for reasons connected with their illness but not due to impaired concentration (see Depression), page 110).

Schizophrenia. The fact that a patient suffers from schizophrenia need not necessarily have any bearing on shoplifting, but in some cases the crime results directly from the illness. The patient may steal as a result of hallucinations instructing him to do so or as a result of delusional belief. Some schizophrenics shoplift quite deliberately in order to obtain the necessities (or indeed the luxuries) of life which their illness makes it difficult for them to earn, while others do so in order to force admission to some form of institution.

In some instances the presence of some mental disorder may be sufficient to make it unlikely that the offender was capable of forming the necessary intent to steal, thus providing a defence against the charge. In many cases it is impossible to determine the degree of intent and the mental state will then be offered in mitigation rather than as a defence.

With regard to depression in relation to shoplifting, it is vital to try and distinguish between pre-existing depression and the reactive depression that most erstwhile respectable ladies will develop when charged with a criminal offence. Thus detailed information from the offender's family doctor should always be obtained, a record of drugs prescribed being an essential part of such information.

Assessment of person charged with 'shoplifting'
In addition to the usual full psychiatric and physical examination, particular attention should be paid to the following aspects:

(1) A detailed history of any preceding or co-existing physical illness.
(2) Detailed enquiry into any medication taken prior to the offence and during the preceding few weeks.

The subject should be specifically asked if he had taken any form of tablets or medicine which he had bought from the chemist or been given by some person other than his family doctor. Many people do not regard patent medicines as being 'drugs' and may fail to mention them if not directly asked. Cold cures are especially important in this respect as many contain antihistamines which can affect the taker's state of awareness. In this context the possible role of alcohol should also be considered as its effects may be potentiated by other drugs.

(3) A detailed account of the offence and the circumstances leading up to it.

Some otherwise perfectly honest people have shoplifted at times of personal crisis. They are not 'confused' in the organic sense, nor 'depressed' in the ill sense, but are suffering from an acute emotional disturbance of a reactive kind. Precipitating events may be anything involving the loss of someone or something dear to the person, or equally the threatened loss of the loved object. Thus shoplifting may be done by the recently bereaved, divorced or separated. It may also occur in people whose relatives are seriously ill, or who are in some form of danger. While not providing a defence such an emotional state may be taken in mitigation.

(4) In those offenders who are thought to be depressed the major difficulty is establishing whether the depression was present at the time of the offence or whether it is a reaction to the arrest.

In addition to taking a detailed chronological history of the development of the depressive disorder from the offender and his relatives, supportive evidence should be sought (with the offender's permission) from the family doctor and any other professional who may have had contact with him. Further supportive evidence may consist of discovering factors which might reasonably be assumed to have precipitated a depressive illness.

Criminal damage

Until 1971 the law covering damage to property was contained in The Malicious Damage Act of 1861. This Act created a large number of offences involving the 'unlawful and malicious' damage of property. In 1970 the Law Commission reported that in their opinion the existing laws were unsatisfactory because of the multiplicity and overlapping of offences, and the variety of penalties. In this report it was recommended that arson—that is damage by fire—should not be a separate crime. However, Parliament decided that because of the special dangers inherent in fire-raising it should remain a specific offence, so the final version of the Criminal Damage Act 1971 contains the following Sections:

Section 1(1)

'A person who without lawful excuse destroys or damages any property belonging to another intending to destroy or damage any such property or being reckless as to whether any such property would be destroyed or damaged shall be guilty of an offence'.

Section 1(2)

'A person who without lawful excuse destroys or damages any property whether belonging to himself or another:
(a) intending to destroy or damage any property or being reckless as to whether any property would be destroyed or damaged; and
(b) intending by the destruction or damage to endanger the life of another or being reckless as to whether the life of another would be thereby endangered shall be guilty of an offence'.

Section 1(3)

'An offence committed under this section by destroying or damaging property by fire shall be charged as arson'.

Not only is the act an offence but threatening to do so is an offence under Section 2 of the Criminal Damage Act 1971.

Section 2

'A person who without lawful excuse makes to another a threat, intending that the other would fear it would be carried out:
(a) to destroy or damage any property belonging to that other or a third person; or
(b) to destroy or damage his own property in a way which he knows is likely to endanger the life of that other or a third person shall be guilty of an offence.'

Mens rea

The requirements of Section 1 (1) are that the destruction or damaging of the property should be intentional or reckless, and without lawful excuse.

Thus the offender must be aware that his conduct involves the risk of damage to the property of another, and that this risk is unjustifiable or unreasonable in the circumstances.

In the case of 'destroying or damaging property with intent to endanger life' there must be a causal relationship between the act causing damage and the endangering of life, and the endangering of life must be intended when the act is committed.

Thus, in such cases, much will depend on the assessment of the intention of the defendant and his capacity at the time to form such an intention.

Taking and driving away (see Chapter 9)

Arson

Arson has always been regarded by the Courts as a most serious crime, partly because of the often immense damage that may occur in financial terms, and more importantly because of the potential risk to life that is inherent in fire-raising. It has not received as much attention from psychiatrists as might be expected, and there is a surprising paucity of literature on the subject.

Social aspects

The cost to the community of fire damage is enormous. The number of cases of arson known to the police has increased steadily from 3,562 cases in 1971 to 9,415 in 1977. Industrial fires alone now cost in the order of fifty million pounds per year. Fires in schools have become a major problem. In considering the question of malicious fire-raising there is obviously a continuum between those who act from clearly defined motives of profit at the one extreme to those psychotic fire-raisers who seem to have no rational reason for so doing at the other. Those people occupying the middle ground of this continuum may present a considerable problem in terms of appropriate management. Those who act for obvious reasons of gain or as part of a political gesture are not primarily the concern of the psychiatrist.

1. Fire-raisers who act for profit
This group is of limited interest to the psychiatrist. The motive is generally financial in that insurance will be collected to a value which exceeds that of the property destroyed. In the U.S.A. professional fire-raisers command high fees for their expert services, but in most cases the fires are started by the owner. It has been said that a number of successful businesses have risen phoenix-like from the ashes of a disastrous fire. At a lower, but no less criminal level, is the housewife who stages a damaging but not dangerous fire in order to have a room refurnished and decorated at the expense of the insurance company.

   Fires are sometimes started in order to destroy evidence of other crimes, particularly murder. A famous case was that of Rouse [2] who wished to disappear and start a fresh life. He gave a lift to a tramp, strangled him and set fire to the car, in the hope that the body would be mistaken for himself.

2. Political fire-raising
This has become an increasingly popular activity amongst revolutionary political parties. The burning of synagogues and the Reichstag in Nazi Germany was the forerunner of the I.R.A.'s present campaign in Northern Ireland.

3. Pathological fire-raisers

(a) *Those with subnormality of intelligence.* At one time arson was regarded as the crime of retarded female adolescents, but the proportion of arsonists who are female has steadily decreased. McKeracher and Dacre's [3] study in 1966 of Subnormal Arsonists in a Special Hospital showed that they differed from the other residents in being less involved in direct physical violence to others and having more psychiatric symptoms.

(b) *Those with organic brain disease.* Occasional cases of fire-raising occurring for the first time in the presence of organic brain disorders have been described. The fire may be started accidentally due to confusion or impaired memory or deliberately as a result of delusional ideas or as part of a general loss of judgement and disinhibition. The possibility of an underlying organic brain disorder should always be considered when fire-raising of a motiveless kind is carried out by someone of previously normal intelligence and personality. In elderly people this is an obvious diagnostic point, but it may be overlooked in younger people.

(c) *Epilepsy* There is no evidence to support the idea that epileptics are prone to fire-raising. In Lewis and Yarnell's [4] series there was no case of postictal arson. It is possible that in rare cases an epileptic might start a fire during a postictal confusional state. Epileptics who do commit arson are much more likely to have done so as a result of personality problems or other psychiatric disorders than due to their epilepsy *per se*.

(d) *Alcoholism.* Alcohol may contribute to fire-raising in several ways. It may be the underlying cause of a dementing illness or a confusional episode as in delirium tremens. It may also act purely as a temporary disinhibiting agent allowing the imbiber to behave in a way which he would control when sober. Alcohol may also be a factor in the development of a delusional state which in turn provokes the fire-raising as a means of getting revenge on those considered to be persecuting the offender.

(e) *Other psychotic disorders.* People suffering from schizophrenia or manic depressive psychosis may start fires. This may be due to hallucinatory instructions or as a result of delusional ideas. In depressed people it may form part of a suicide attempt or a suicide plus homicide. In mania, fire-raising may occur as part of the grandiose notions held by the sufferer, but more often it is due to the underlying hostility and aggression demonstrated by many hypomanics.

4. Non-psychotic fire-raisers

There are many fire-raisers in whom no evidence of psychotic illness can be demonstrated, and yet who act from motives which seem irrational or inadequate to the observer. While there is often more than one motive operating within the individual, it is possible to sub-divide this group on the basis of their stated motives.

(a) *Revenge.* This sub-group merges into the morbidly jealous or persecuted but some individuals act as a result of a genuine grievance such as being sacked or jilted by their lover. Their reaction is disproportionate to the injury they have sustained and may reflect either their excessively aggressive personality or their paranoid attitudes. The nature of their underlying personality can be demonstrated by their response to a wide variety of life experiences.

(b) *Heroism.* Some fire-raisers act as a way of becoming the centre of attention. Having started a blaze they summon the fire brigade, help rescue people and generally try to be centre stage. Occasionally, a member of the fire service acts in this way.

(c) *A cry for help.* Very rarely someone in a state of desperation draws attention to their plight by starting a fire. This usually follows some acute crisis in that person's life, such as bereavement, divorce or other separation.

(d) *Sexually motivated fire-raising.* Several studies [5, 6] have shown that arsonists show a greater degree of sexual problems than other offenders. These studies were, however, on arsonists confined in prisons or special hospitals.

A small number of fire-raisers have a fetish about fire. This may start as an association between staring into a fire and fantasising pictures while masturbating. Gradually the need for bigger and better blazes takes over and the offender moves from relatively harmless fires to starting serious conflagrations. The fetish fire-raiser tends to select occupied buildings and thus is highly dangerous.

Some offenders while not deriving direct sexual excitement from watching a fire may use the technique as a way of reassuring themselves about their potency and virility. Such offenders are likely to be sexually inadequate and under achievers in other fields of endeavour.

(e) *Children as fire-raisers.* Several studies of child fire-raisers have been carried out [7, 8, 9]. In some children it seems to represent an exaggeration of the normal experimental and exploratory behaviour, but in others it appears to be part of a more seriously disturbed behaviour pattern. Such children come from homes characterised by severe parental psychopathology. According to Vandersal [9] such children showed—'a sense of exclusion, loneliness and unfilled dependency needs'. Many of the children also showed learning difficulties and had failed at school. There may be a link between fire-raising and the presence of minimal brain damage. In many instances fire-raising seems to help the child derive relief from some overpowering anxiety.

Female arsonists
Arson is predominantly a male crime (about 85%) but women fire-raisers can be just as dangerous as their male counterparts. Tennent et al [10] examined female arsonists in three special hospitals and compared them to a matched group of non-fire-raisers. Less than half of the arson group had actually been prosecuted for arson which suggests that it is not as uncommon a crime in women as official figures show. The study showed that separation from parents occurred significantly more often in arsonists than controls in the period before the age of three. In general arsonists appeared to have more problems related to their sexual relationships than the control group. In respect of previous psychiatric symptomatology, age of first psychiatric contact and mean length of hospitalisation, there were no significant differences between the two groups.

Assessment in cases of arson

As in any serious crime, the Court will be concerned with the likelihood of further offences. The recidivist element in arson may well have been exaggerated in the past. Soothill's 20-year cohort study showed that the vast majority were not reconvicted for arson [11]. It is, therefore, even more important to try and detect those few who are likely to re-offend in order that they are prevented from so doing, while others are not unnecessarily detained. While it is obviously impossible to be sure in any individual case, the following factors have some predictive value:

1. A history of previous fire-raising
This must extend beyond actual previous convictions for arson as many such events are not detected or cannot be brought to court for lack of evidence. Fire-raising may also not be prosecuted as arson *per se* but as

wilful damage. Hence a detailed examination of records may be required as well as a patient enquiry as to past behaviour from the offender and close relatives. Anyone may commit arson on one occasion, but when they repeat it a second time the chances of further offences becomes very much greater.

2. Evidence of psychopathic personality

A history of being repeatedly at odds with those in authority, of having poor control over impulsive behaviour and general difficulty in relationships suggests a greater likelihood of recidivism. This is even more likely if the individual also abuses alcohol in a regular or intermittent way.

3. The social situation of the individual

The greater the degree of isolation that exists between the offender and society at large, the greater the risk of repeated offences. Those who offend at a time when their normal social links have been disrupted for some reason are less likely to offend again if new contacts are made and fresh supportive relationships established. In considering the offence it is important to look at the ways in which the offender's life situation has been altered by the act.

4. What were the underlying motives?

In many instances the motives must remain a matter of speculation, but in some cases they may be expressed quite clearly. In cases where the motive is the obtaining of sexual gratification or even the relief of tension through fire-raising, the risk of further fire-setting is high.

5. Is there evidence of mental disorder?

The presence of subnormality of intelligence in addition to the above factors increases the risk of repetition. While some people commit arson only as a result of suffering from a specific episode of mental illness they form a small part of the total group. A large percentage of arsonists however have a history of previous psychiatric symptoms and psychiatric treatment unrelated to their offence.

References

Offences against property

Shoplifting
1   Gibbens, T C N, Palmer, C and Prince, J (1971) Mental health aspects of shoplifting. *British Medical Journal*, **3**, 612–615

Arson
2 Rouse A A (1952) *Notable British Trials Series* (Ed) Helena Normanton. William Hodge & Co. Ltd., Glasgow
3 McKeracher, D W and Dacre, A J I (1966) *British Journal of Psychiatry*, **112**, 1151–1154
4 Lewis, N D S and Yarnell, H (1951) Pathological Firesetting. Nervous & Mental Diseases Monograph, No. 82. New York
5 Lewis N D S and Yarnell, H, *Ibid*
6 Tennent, T G, McQuaid A and Hands, N J (1971) *British Journal of Psychiatry*, **119**, 497–502
7 Lewis, N D S and Yarnell, H, *Ibid*
8 Bender, L (1953) Firesetting in Children. In: *Aggression, Hostility and Anxiety in Children*. Charles C Thomas, Springfield, Illinois
9 Vandersal, T A and Weiner, J M (1970) *Archives of General Psychiatry*, **22**, 63–71
10 Tennent, T G et al, *Op. cit.*
11 Soothill, K L and Pope, P J (1973) *Medicine, Science and the Law*, **13** (2) 127–138

Further reading

Scott, D (1974) *Fire and Fire-raisers*. Duckworth, London
Fry, J F and Le Couter, N B (1966) Arson. *Medico-Legal Journal*, **xxxiv**, 108–121
Inciardi, J (1970) The adult firesetter—a typology. *Criminology*, **8** (2), 145-155
Macht, L B and Mack, J E (1968) The firesetter syndrome. *Psychiatry*, **31**, 277–288
Harley, W P and Monahan, T M (1969) *British Journal of Criminology*, **9**, 4
Scott, D (1977) Malicious fire-raising. *Practitioner*, **218** (1308), 812–817
Scott, D (1978) The problems of malicious fire-raising. *British Journal of Hospital Medicine*, **19** (3), 259–263
Prins, H A (1978) Their candles are all out . . . or are they? *Royal Society of Health Journal*, Aug.

9. Road Traffic Offences

Current legislation is embodied in the Road Traffic Act of 1972. The main provisions include:

(1) Causing death by reckless or dangerous driving

'A person who causes the death of another person by the driving of a motor vehicle on a road recklessly, or at a speed or in a manner which is dangerous to the public, having regard to all the circumstances of the case, including the nature, condition and use of the road, and the amount of traffic which is actually at the time, or which might reasonably be expected to be, on the road, shall be guilty of an offence.' (Section 1 (1))

(2) Reckless and dangerous driving

'If a person drives a motor vehicle on a road recklessly or at a speed or in a manner which is dangerous to the public . . . he shall be guilty of an offence.' (Section 2)

(3) Careless and inconsiderate driving

'If a person drives a motor vehicle on a road without due care and attention, or without reasonable consideration for other persons using the road, he shall be guilty of an offence.'

The relevance of the above offences to forensic psychiatry is that there may be a defence to the charge if the accused can show that he suffered a sudden change in consciousness for which he was not to blame. This is in effect the defence of automatism. The legal definition of non-insane automatism is:

'An act done by the muscles without any control by the mind such as a spasm, a reflex action or a convulsion, or an act done by a person who is not conscious of what he is doing, such as an act done whilst suffering from concussion or whilst sleep walking.' (Denning [1])

Although not included in this definition altered consciousness caused by hypoglycaemia has been regarded as 'non-insane automatism'. In these cases the accused bears only an 'evidential burden'. He must introduce evidence from which it may be reasonably concluded that his actions at the time of the alleged offence were involuntary. The accused's own statement will rarely be sufficient unless supported by adequate medical evidence (see Hypoglycaemia, page 131).

Driving while unfit

'A person, who, when driving, or attempting to drive a motor vehicle on a road or other public place, is unfit to drive through drink or drugs, shall be guilty of an offence'. (Section 5 (1))

'A person, who, when in charge of a motor vehicle on a road or other public place, is unfit to drive through drink or drugs, is guilty of an offence'. (Section 5 (2))

Evidence of unfitness to drive may include the proportion or quantity of alcohol or other drug in the blood or body of the accused, as ascertained by analysis of a specimen taken from him with his consent.

A person who, without reasonable excuse, fails to provide a specimen for a laboratory test is guilty of an offence.

A person who 'drives or attempts to drive a motor vehicle on a road or other public place, having consumed alcohol in such a quantity that the proportion in his blood, as ascertained from a laboratory test for which he subsequently provides a specimen, exceeds the prescribed limit at the time he provides the specimen, shall be guilty of an offence'.

The present prescribed limit means 80 mg of alcohol in 100 ml of blood.

The psychiatrist may be involved in cases of unfitness to drive in a number of ways. First, he may be asked to give evidence on behalf of a person who claims to have some neurological or psychiatric conditions which might cause the layman to regard him as being drunk. Second, he may be asked to assess whether or not the offender has an alcoholic problem in which case the Court may wish to make some recommendations in respect of treatment. Third, he may be asked his view on whether the drugs a patient is taking may render him unfit to drive, or if a combination of such drugs with alcohol under the prescribed limit would lead to unfitness. Finally, the psychiatrist may be asked to comment on the fitness to drive of someone suffering from some mental disorder, or some form of epilepsy.

There is little evidence to suggest that a functional psychotic illness increases the likelihood of having an accident, with the exceptions of illnesses in which the sufferer has symptoms related to motoring. Examples being the depressed patient who takes suicidal risks as a way of killing himself without it necessarily being regarded as suicide, or the schizophrenic who has delusions regarding other drivers persecuting him.

Presenile dementias may present as the result of motoring accidents occurring before anyone has recognised other symptoms in the patient. Such accidents may arise from failure of concentration, or as a result of spatial disorientation leading to dangerous indecision.

Personality disorders are over-represented in those having traffic accidents. Studies have shown that hospitalised psychopaths had twice as many previous accidents as any other diagnostic group [2].

Alcoholics, naturally, have a high risk both of dangerous driving charges and driving under the influence.

The driving of heavy goods vehicles and public service vehicles demands even higher standards of physical and mental fitness. People who have suffered a psychotic illness should not drive such vehicles.

Drivers who develop symptoms of mental illness should be laid off work without delay. Those who require continuing psychotropic medication should not continue in this type of work.

Drugs and driving

The greatest danger is in the early stages of taking a new drug or combination of drugs before the individual has developed any degree of tolerance to the drug and before he has had time to assess any possible side effects.

A large number of people driving at any time in this country are on some form of psychotrophic drug. Such people are also likely, at times, to combine these drugs with alcohol.

The most commonly prescribed drugs are anxyolitic agents, mainly those belonging to the diazepam group. While small doses have not been shown to impair driving ability, their concurrent use with alcohol may do so, having a multiplying rather than a purely additive effect.

The major tranquillisers such as the phenothiazines and butyrophe-
nones have a certain amount of sedative action, and their effect on
driving is likely to be proportionate to this effect. Loomis (1962) [3]
demonstrated quite marked impairment with small doses of chlorpro-
mazine.

Antidepressants—tricyclics
Most of these drugs cause drowsiness in a proportion of patients,
particularly during the first few days of treatment. They are also apt to
cause blurring of vision. They should not be combined with alcohol.

Monoamine oxidase inhibitors
The main danger with these drugs is the onset of a hypertensive crisis
due to reaction with other drugs or food substances.

Anaesthetic agents
Many have relatively long half-lives and can continue to interfere with
driving skills for many hours after they have been administered.

Taking and driving away

This offence is actually an offence against property but as the offender
is often not qualified to drive, and is always uninsured at the time, there
are usually additional road traffic offences on the charge. Car thefts in
which the primary intention is not to deprive the owner permanently of
his car, but merely to 'borrow' it, are one of the major nuisances of
urban living.

There are a number of different forms of car stealing, though there is
obviously a degree of overlap between the groups.

(1) Professional thefts—the type of car is carefully selected and its
    appearance and registration numbers rapidly changed to enable
    it to be re-sold.
(2) Thefts in order to steal the contents of the vehicle or to use it in
    some other criminal activity.
(3) Joy riding—this is probably the most common form and is
    usually perpetrated by a group of youths who feel they need a
    car for a few hours, abandoning it when they have achieved
    their goal or it runs out of petrol.

(4) Repetitive thefts by youths with an overwhelming desire to drive and a fascination for cars.

Though groups 3 and 4 are of interest from the psychiatric point of view, they have received relatively little attention.

There does not seem to be a clear consensus of opinion as to the dangerousness of these groups of drivers. The major factor, as with ordinary owner-drivers, seems to be the level of blood alcohol. Many car thieves are undetected unless stopped for coincidental offences, hence such offences are over-represented in those charged. The majority of offenders sentenced for taking and driving away are disqualified from driving, so that if they re-offend, they are additionally guilty of driving while disqualified. In some cases disqualification makes rehabilitation more difficult, because the normal channels for satisfying their urge to drive cars are closed to them.

Gibbens [4] studied 39 boys who had committed motor vehicle offences and been sent to Borstal. He compared them to a similar group who had committed non-vehicular offences and found that they differed in a number of characteristics. They tended to be boys from 'intact' homes, often the later members of large families, who were sent to Borstal after several convictions for which they had not received custodial sentences. They were no less seriously delinquent than the rest, and their prognosis was no better.

Gibbens suggested that the crime often had a symbolic significance and tended to be unconsciously motivated. The motives were often multi-factorial, and included a search for excitement, and a demonstration of masculinity. He commented on a small sub-group in whom the offence seemed to be much more 'neurotic' in that the criminal activity was repetitive and near compulsive. The boys involved often had close relationships with a dominant mother and their father seemed to play little part in the life of the family.

References

Road traffic offences

1 Denning (1963) Bratty *v* Attorney-General for Northern Ireland
2 Eclkema, R C et al (1970) A statistical study on the relationship between mental illness and traffic accidents. *American Journal of Public Health*, **60**, 459–469

3 Loomis T A (1963) Effects of alcohol on persons using tranquillisers. *Proceedings of the 3rd International Conference on Alcohol and Road Traffic*, page 119. British Medical Association, London

Further reading

Medical Aspects of Fitness to Drive, 3rd edition, 1976. Medical Commission on Accident Prevention

Taking and driving away

4 Gibbens, T C N (1958) *British Journal of Delinquency*, **8**, 257–265

Further reading

Willet, T C (1964) *Criminal on the Road*. Tavistock Publications, London

Part 3 Psychiatric Syndromes in Relation to Crime

10. Affective Disorders

While there is continuing debate concerning the classification of affective disorders it is sufficient for the purpose of this book to divide the conditions in the traditional way into reactive depression, endogenous depression, hypomania and mania. In all cases the primary change is an alteration in mood, and it is this which gives rise to the symptoms. An individual in his lifetime may demonstrate various sequences or combinations of these affective changes. The following patterns may be observed in an individual's history:

(1) A single depressive episode.
(2) A single manic episode.
(3) Recurrent depressive episodes.
(4) Recurrent manic episodes.
(5) Circular psychoses—i.e., episodes of both manic and depression at different time.
(6) Mixed affective states.

Additionally, individuals may show fluctuations in mood which do not amount to full scale manic or depressive episodes. This is referred to as cyclothymia. Other people appear to have a permanently raised mood and are described as having hyperthymia. While manic depressive disorders are more common in people of cyclothymic personality they are not exclusive to this group, nor does everyone of that type of personality develop an affective illness during their life.

The attempt to distinguish between reactive and endogenous depression can be extremely difficult if not impossible in some cases. In clinical practice cases are frequently met in which the symptoms are suggestive of a reactive depression, yet no precipitating factor can be uncovered. In other cases which start as a reactive depression to an obvious stress, the symptom pattern changes after some time, and is then clinically indistinguishable from the so-called endogenous type. Finally, some individuals have recurrent episodes of depression which always present with the endogenous constellation of symptoms but which sometimes clearly follow a 'depressing' experience while at other times seem to occur without any external cause.

In forensic psychiatry the main reason for trying to distinguish between the two kinds of depression is that the psychiatrist is asked to see the person *after* he has been charged with an offence, and it is important to decide whether any symptoms of depression are due to the new circumstances or whether they predate the commission of the crime. It is important to remember, however, that someone with a reactive depression may commit a crime because of his mood state just as much as someone suffering from an endogenous disorder.

Reactive depression

The sufferer tends to feel more depressed as the day goes by, and often has difficulty in getting to sleep. He is able to respond to some extent to cheerful company and generally blames external events for his problems rather than expressing ideas of personal guilt. There may be an underlying anger and resentment. Delusional ideas are not expressed.

Endogenous depression

The clinical picture varies depending to some extent on the individual's basic personality, and in some cases on the age of the sufferer. The mood is low and the sufferer feels gloomy and despondent. Though many are tearful some feel as if they have 'gone beyond tears' and say that it would be a relief to cry. Their general level of interest, activity and enthusiasm is low so that they describe how they no longer enjoy things which once gave them pleasure and how even small problems present as being insoluble. Their level of physical activity may be greatly reduced, in some cases to the point of stupor. Those who are anxious as well as depressed may however present with restlessness and agitation, constantly seeking reassurance which when given only briefly helps. In this setting of misery life is seen as unrewarding and burdensome so that the idea of death becomes attractive and suicide may be contemplated or attempted.

In severe depressive conditions the patient may develop delusional ideas. These usually fall into one or more of the following categories:

(1) Delusion of guilt and unworthiness.
(2) Delusions of poverty.
(3) Nihilistic delusions.
(4) Hypochondriacal delusions.
(5) Paranoid delusions.

Sleep is generally disturbed, typically with early waking, but all variations may occur. The morning is usually the worst time and the sufferer may lie awake in the early hours dreading the coming day. Concentration is impaired because of a tendency to revert to morbid preoccupations. Decisions are made with difficulty and having dithered for a long time the sufferer may finally act in what seems to be an impulsive and inappropriate manner without apparently realising the consequence of his actions.

The crimes that may be committed by someone in a depressed state reflect some of the symptoms of the illness. Thus, some depressed people seem to be unable to seek help by a conventional approach to their doctor and attempt to draw attention to their plight by some gesture which may have a self destructive element in it. The most common gesture is an attempted suicide and the 'cry for help' aspect of such a gesture is well recognised. Some people substitute shoplifting for suicide, which though not life threatening can be very destructive to their reputation and standing in the community. It also has the added advantage of embarrassing relatives who may not have been sufficiently attentive to the needs of the offender.

Suicide may itself be accompanied by the killing of the nearest and dearest because of the depressive's reluctance to leave them facing the hostile world alone. Homicide may occur also as a result of paranoid ideas which lead the offender to believe that his suffering is due to the malignant influence of the victim.

Any well publicised crime, particularly if it is violent or bizarre, will attract confessions from people who are in fact totally innocent. Some, at least, of these will be depressives whose ideas of guilt and unworthiness lead them to accept the blame. Usually they can easily be eliminated from inquiries but occasionally they may seem highly likely suspects and waste a great deal of time and effort on the part of the police.

Shoplifting has been mentioned as a possible cry for help, but it may also arise through preoccupation and a failure to concentrate. This is particularly likely in the case of a young woman with post-natal depression who may be harassed in her shopping by the demands of an older toddler. It also occurs in elderly depressives in whom the situation may be worsened by tranquillising drugs prescribed for their apparent anxiety, but which do nothing for the underlying depression.

Arson is occasionally committed by depressed people as part of a suicide attempt.

Murder by depressives is generally restricted to the killing of close relatives and is often followed by the suicide of the offender. Infanticide and the killing of older children by their mother is sometimes due to a post-natal depression and the risk of this happening should always be taken into account when treating a depressed mother with small children. Assaults by mothers on their children which do not result in the death of the child may also be symptomatic of a depressive illness in the mother.

Mania and hypomania

The difference between hypomania and mania is one of degree. The hypomanic is mildly or moderately overactive. There is a loss of inhibition and the mood varies from an elation to one of angry excitement. There may be marked irritability and aggression. The sufferer is overactive, flitting from one activity to another, speech is increased and shows flight of ideas and distractability. His ideas may not show logical connections, being influenced by chance events in this environment, or even the sounds and associations of the words he is using.

Some will express delusional ideas which may be grandiose in content. Their disinhibited comments about those around them may provoke angry reactions which in turn convince them that people are against them. Sometimes they have erotic notions about comparative strangers and may act on what they imagine is a sexual invitation— much to the alarm of the innocent victim.

Crimes committed by hypomanic or manic individuals include crimes of violence due to the loss of control, irritability and lack of judgement. Crimes of fraud, false pretences and the like may result from the grandiose notions or delusions.

Some hypomanics are given to taking and driving away other people's cars, or test driving new cars which they fail to return to the garage.

Those who develop delusions about their own importance may commit crimes in the belief that they are 'King' or 'God', and are entitled to behave in whatever way they choose.

The management of offenders in whom there is a clear causal link between the offence and an affective illness should primarily be directed at the treatment of the underlying disorder. It may be that at least in the initial stage such treatment is best carried out in a setting of reasonable security not only for the protection of the public, but also to protect the sufferer from the possibility of inflicting harm on himself.

11. Schizophrenia

People suffering from a schizophrenic disorder may commit any form of crime without their illness having any direct bearing on their offence, though the Court may take their illness into account when deciding on disposal. A schizophrenic illness may be causally related to a criminal act in a number of ways. It is convenient to consider these under the broad headings of positive and negative symptoms. Positive symptoms are those which are present during active phases of the illness and diminish to a greater or lesser degree during remissions. In some patients they vanish completely during remission, in others they persist in spite of all treatment. The negative or deficit symptoms are much harder to define. They are regarded as the scarring of the personality produced by the active disease, though in some instances they may be the result of institutionalisation or social isolation.

'Positive' symptoms

Hallucinations

A common symptom in schizophrenic illness is auditory hallucinations. These are often of an accusatory or derogatory nature. Sufferers are sometimes provoked into assaults on people whom they consider to be the source of these voices. The victim may be totally unknown to the perpetrator and the crime may seem to be totally spontaneous and lacking in motive. The victim may, however, be a significant figure in the offender's life, and may well have given him some basis for his feelings of persecution in which case the offender may seem to have a relatively normal motive for the offence.

Hallucinations may take the form of instructions to the sufferer which he may find difficult to ignore. Acting on such instructions the individual may assault innocent bystanders. Cases have occurred of a person being pushed under an approaching tube train by a complete stranger on the basis of such 'instructions'. Instructions of this kind can lead to crimes of theft as well as offences against the person.

Delusions

Delusions of persecution are relatively common in schizophrenic disorders, particularly in the so-called paranoid group. The delusions may be ill-formed and generalised, or they may be related to the imagined wrongdoing of a specific individual. In the former, the sufferer may make an unprovoked attack on anyone he feels is connected with his persecutors, while in the latter, the attack will be directed at the identified individual. People in public office are especially prone to attracting this kind of attention. The behaviour may be confined to the sending of threatening or offensive letters, but such threats should not be idly dismissed as they may be the forewarnings of a serious attack.

Grandiose delusions sometimes occur in schizophrenia and may also be the direct cause of criminal behaviour. The sufferer may believe that he is omnipotent and has the right to do anything he chooses. This may include taking the life of a lesser being or appropriating anything he wants to his own use.

Thought disorder

The capacity for logical, goal-directed thinking may be impaired and in some instances can lead to behaviour which the outsider would regard as bizarre but which makes some kind of sense to the schizophrenic. The fact that the motive for the crime lacks any ordinary sense does not imply that the crime itself will not be carried out with cunning. There may be considerable method to the madness. This aspect has given rise to great confusion in lawyers who seem to find it difficult to conceive that someone can be extremely mentally disordered and yet behave for much of the time in a perfectly normal fashion.

'Negative' symptoms

Symptoms such as apathy, volitional defect, affective flattening, lack of social judgement, have been variously ascribed to the schizophrenic process, and to the treatment or lack of treatment which the sufferer has received. Whatever the cause there is no doubt that there are a substantial number of people who are only at times actively psychotic but who are at best socially and personally inadequate. Such people used to form the more or less permanent sub-culture of the mental hospital back wards, but having been subjected to considerable therapeutic zeal may have been discharged to community care (more accurately, community 'couldn't care less'). For a while this stage army occupied many of the beds provided for the homeless and destitute by charitable organisations. Since many of these establishments have been converted into hotels for foreign tourists, the social flotsam has ebbed and flowed between prison, doss house and the more tolerant mental hospitals. The crimes they commit are often petty, but the sentences they attract may be severe because of the apparently appalling record of convictions they have. Imprisonment merely increases their dependence and institutionalisation, to say nothing of overwhelming the prisons and preventing them doing the work for which they were established.

It is important to remember that serious crimes committed by schizophrenics are rare. They tend to attract undue attention because of the sometimes bizarre circumstances surrounding them. Schizophrenia is a relatively common condition and the vast majority of those who suffer from it represent no problem of criminal behaviour.

Hallucinations

An hallucination is a sensory perception arising in the absence of an external stimulus. Thus it differs from an illusion which is an incorrect perception of an actual stimulus. Attempts have been made to distinguish 'true' hallucinations from other related forms of mental imagery, but no totally successful scheme has been evolved.

Under normal conditions, the brain is constantly receiving a vast amount of sensory input both from the external and internal world. This material is filtered and selected so that certain stimuli are acted upon consciously or unconsciously, but both selected and unselected stimuli contribute to the general state of arousal of the brain. Hallucinations may be provoked by localised stimuli to the cortex, or by general factors affecting the alerting pathways of the reticulo-hypothalamic-thalamic system.

Hallucinations are of forensic importance in two ways. First they may provoke the offender into committing a criminal act, and secondly their presence suggests the possibility of a mental disorder which may be relevant, even though there is no direct link between the hallucination itself and the crime.

Hallucinations may occur in the normal person, particularly at times when the level of consciousness is changing, i.e. when waking or when going to sleep.

Hallucinations may arise as a result of damage to the peripheral sensory organs, phantom limb phenomena being an obvious example.

Conditions of sensory deprivation may produce hallucinatory experiences in people without evidence of any mental or physical illness. Such conditions may be deliberately induced as part of an attempt at brain-washing, but can also arise unintentionally during forms of medical treatment involving tank respirators.

Hallucinations are a frequent symptom in temporal lobe epilepsy and may involve a number of sensory modalities. They may be highly complex experiences in which previous events or situations in the sufferer's life are re-lived, or they may be relatively simple single sense hallucinations, such as bangs, clicks or whistling noises. The hallucinations are often accompanied by specific emotional experiences. The nature of the hallucination may help localise the lesion, but in some instances can be misleading.

Hallucinations may arise in any form of brain disorder due to structural or physiological damage. In general purely visual hallucinations tend to indicate organic brain disorder; while pure auditory hallucinations are more common in the 'functional' illnesses. It is these auditory hallucinations which are the most likely to lead directly to criminal acts.

Hallucinations are relatively common in schizophrenic disorders and were regarded by Schneider [1] as being of primary importance in the diagnosis of such disorders. He included in his first rank symptoms auditory hallucinations of the following types:

(1) Voices which repeat or anticipate the patient's own thoughts (echo de penseé or Gedankenlautwerden).
(2) Voices which discuss the patient or argue about him, referring to him in the third person.
(3) Voices discussing the patient's thoughts or behaviour as if giving a running commentary on him.

Hallucinatory voices (phenomes) are the form most likely to provoke criminal acts. These may be the result of the voices issuing specific instructions to carry out some act, an act which may be regarded both by the sufferer and those who know him as totally foreign to his nature.

Some schizophrenics attribute the voices to actual people and assault that person because of the imagined insults. This may lead to totally unexpected and unprovoked assaults on people known to the perpetrator or on complete strangers.

Simple auditory hallucinations occur in schizophrenia and in organic psychosis. With the exception of temporal lobe disturbances, elaborate phenomes are uncommon in organic states.

Occasionally phenomes occur in depressive states, usually taking the form of critical comments or instructions to kill himself. Unlike the schizophrenic, the depressive tends to feel that the comments are justified as they fit in with his own notions of guilt and unworthiness.

Hallucinations may form a prominent feature of syndromes which involve clouding of consciousness. In such cases, auditory hallucinations are almost always restricted to noises or music, and visual hallucinations are more prominent. The visual hallucination may be simple (flashes of light, coloured objects), or they may be complicated visions. In states of delirium the visual hallucinations tend to be terrifying and the sufferer may respond by aggressive behaviour in an attempt to escape.

In organic states, hallucinations of touch are not uncommon, and usually take the form of feeling insects or other animals creeping over the skin. Such symptoms are sometimes a feature of cocaine psychosis.

Sexual hallucinations are a variety of tactile hallucinations though it is often difficult to distinguish between hallucinations and delusions. Such experiences may be reported by schizophrenics, and they may interpret them as rape. The psychotic nature of such complaints is usually revealed by the impossible and bizarre nature of the interference. Not every schizophrenic who complains of sexual interference is hallucinated or deluded!

Hallucinations of smell occur in temporal lobe epilepsy, often as part of the aura of an attack. Schizophrenics sometimes complain of being able to smell poisonous gases or they may believe that they can smell something unpleasant emanating from themselves.

Delusional states

There are few topics in psychiatry which create greater confusion and disagreement than the classification of disorders which are dominated by delusional ideas. There are areas of general agreement such as the delusions associated with depressive disorders, or those arising in organic brain disease, but there is a large grey area in which labels such as paranoia, paranoid personality, paranoid reaction states, and even paranoid schizophrenia are applied in a somewhat arbitrary fashion. The nosological uncertainty reflects the present ignorance regarding the aetiology and pathology of these conditions. At present there is no satisfactory system of classification, yet in order to clarify consideration of a particular individual some nosological framework is necessary.

The first difficulty is to achieve a satisfactory definition of a delusion and to distinguish it from related phenomena. The following types of phenomena are generally described:

Delusional idea

A false belief which is held, in spite of proof to the contrary, and which is not in keeping with the person's educational, social and religious background.

Delusional ideas are divided into primary and secondary delusions. Primary delusions being those which arise *de novo* and cannot be understood in terms of the patient's previous personality experiences, or mood state. Secondary delusions are those which can be understood in terms of some other psychological event.

Some delusional ideas arise as a result of what have been called primary delusional experiences. A number of such experiences can be distinguished, the more important of these being:

(1) The delusional mood
This is a strange mood in which the sufferer feels that the environment has changed in some indefinable but threatening way. As a consequence he feels tense, anxious and perplexed. Such a mood may gradually fade away or it may resolve in the sufferer developing a sudden delusional idea, or having a delusional perception.

(2) Delusional perception
This is a normal perception which is suddenly endowed with a special meaning or significance for the person without rational or emotional cause. In the absence of organic brain disorder, delusional perceptions are usually regarded as being pathognomonic of schizophrenia.

(3) Over-valued ideas

Over-valued ideas may be true but they attract a disproportionate affective investment on the part of the person holding them. They are understandable in terms of the holder's personality, past experience or present situation. They may distort the holder's judgement of reality as much as if they were delusional ideas.

The importance of delusional disorders from the medicolegal point of view is:

(a) The crime is a direct result of the delusional belief held by the offender.

(b) While the crime is not directly related to the delusional ideas, the presence of such beliefs is symptomatic of a disorder which may be relevant in terms of the offender's culpability, or in deciding an appropriate disposal.

In cases where the crime has arisen as a result of the offender acting out his delusional beliefs and committing homicide, the possibility of the defence of insanity (McNaughton Rules) or of diminished responsibility may be raised.

In examining a person who expresses delusional ideas it is important to pay attention both to the form and content of the delusion and also to the total circumstances in which it is occurring. In ordinary clinical practice it may on occasions be possible to identify potentially dangerous situations and by appropriate treatment avoid the commission of a crime.

Content of delusions

Paranoid delusions

This general term is often used as if it meant only persecutory delusions but it includes delusions in which the person falsely believes he is the subject of special attention from other people. Thus it includes not only ideas of persecution but also delusions of reference and grandiose delusions.

Persecutory delusions

This type of delusional ideation is obviously of considerable importance as a motive in violent crimes and probably accounts for the majority of psychotic killings outside the family setting. The greatest risk arises in cases where the 'persecution' is seen as being due to the action of a particular individual rather than a group or organisation, and where the delusions are accompanied by considerable affective loading.

Persecutory delusions are found in schizophrenia, hypomania, depression, organic states and personality disorders.

Grandiose delusions

The sufferer may believe that he is a person of great importance or that he is related to such people. He may believe that he possesses some vitally important secret, or that he has the capacity for influencing affairs of state. As a result of these ideas he may feel that he is being persecuted by other people. Some people with delusions of grandeur may believe that they are 'above the law' and consider themselves entitled to act in whatever way they choose.

Such delusions may occur in schizophrenia, hypomania and in organic states. Classically they were said to occur in General Paralysis of the Insane (G.P.I) though only a minority of such patients showed this type of delusion.

Hypochondriacal delusions

Delusions that one is suffering from a serious disease rarely give rise to criminal offences though they not infrequently lead to suicide, particularly in the elderly. Occasionally, a person convinced that he or she is suffering from an illness which is inherited or transmitted in some other way may kill his or her offspring to spare them future suffering, or kill the person they feel is responsible for their own illness.

Hypochondriacal delusions are most common in depressive disorders but also occur in schizophrenia and in personality disorders.

Delusions of guilt and unworthiness

The person may be convinced that he has committed some crime for which he deserves punishment and for which there can be no forgiveness. Another may believe that he has failed all those whom he loves and that he has brought pain and suffering upon them. Such ideas may be accompanied by a great sense of hopelessness. Such delusions may lead to suicide attempts and in some instances such attempts will be preceded by the killing of those people who are dependent on the sufferer. Ideas of this kind, particularly when accompanied by statements that the world is a wicked and dangerous place, should be viewed seriously especially when the person is living with a spouse and young children.

Delusions of poverty
The false belief that one is poverty-stricken is more likely to lead to suicidal behaviour than any criminal act. However, this type of delusion is most commonly seen in depressive illness and is often only one of a number of other delusional ideas of the types described above.

Morbid jealousy (delusions of infidelity)
This variety of delusional belief is of special forensic interest because of its association with murder. Jealousy is an emotion which arises when one is troubled by the belief, suspicion, or fear that someone one desires for oneself has been, or is about to be, taken from one by another. It is an emotion which everyone experiences at some time or another. Such 'normal' or 'reactive' jealousy shades into excessive possessiveness and from that into morbid or psychotic jealousy in which the sufferer is convinced in a delusional way of the infidelity of the loved one.

States of morbid jealousy have provided the material for a number of literary masterpieces of which Shakespeare's 'Othello' is the best known. The subject has also attracted the attention of a number of psychiatrists. In 1910 Jaspers [2] wrote a paper on Morbid Jealousy in which he suggested there were three main ways in which morbid jealousy might arise. First, it could develop as an understandable progression in a person who had always shown progressive and paranoid traits. Secondly, it could arise as a direct change in the personality, something new and alien, which he attributed to a pathological 'process'. Thirdly, he described cases in which it had arisen as part of an organic brain disorder. Most subsequent writers have employed similar divisions. Todd and Dewhurst [3] suggested the title 'Othello Syndrome' should be applied to those cases where the delusions of infidelity occurred in pure form, not in the setting of an already established psychosis. Mowat [4], in his study of 'Morbid Jealousy and Murder', showed that almost half of those who at the time of the murder showed only delusions of infidelity, later developed other signs suggestive of schizophrenia.

There would seem, however, to be a certain number of people in whom the morbid jealousy remains constant and free from other psychotic symptomatology. In Mowat's [4] study there were 40 male murderers; 13 were adjudged to be schizophrenic, 8 depressive, 6 alcoholic and 2 had organic illnesses. He was able to describe a 'typical' case history of a murder due to morbid jealousy.

'Usually during the early years of the marriage the man is not jealous, but after some six years or so he begins to feel that his wife no longer cares for him. He soon becomes convinced that she is unfaithful and finds 'evidence' to support his belief. In a curious way, however, he often avoids unequivocal proof of his suspicions. His evidence is often contradictory and inconsistent. He spends hours interrogating his spouse, trying to get her to confess. These sessions often lead to rows and violence. This in turn may lead to his wife leaving him, only to be persuaded to return by promises and protestations. The scope of his delusional ideas increases and he believes that he has caught VD from her, or that their children are not really his. Finally, in his late 40s, having been deluded for four or five years, he kills her by strangulation, or by clubbing her to death.'*

The psychopathology of this condition is complicated and varied, but in general there is a basic feeling of inferiority which renders the sufferer vulnerable to real or imagined threats from those whom he conceives of as being more potent or powerful than himself.

In some cases the spouse is regarded primarily as a possession, so that any signs of increased independence on her part will be seen as a threat, as will any signs of interest shown her by other men.

In some cases, the inadequacy arises from the sufferer's own problems of fidelity, either in the past or desired in the future. These problems are then projected on to the spouse and on to the males with whom she comes in contact.

In other cases, the inadequacy stems from actual failures at sexual performance, or from exaggerated notions as to how others perform. This form of inadequacy is often seen in cases of morbid jealousy associated with alcoholism. It is not always clear whether the impotence is a result of 'Brewer's droop' or whether the drinking problem arises from the fear of impotence, real or imagined. In Mowat's series, only 12% of male murderers had problems of impotence prior to the crime.

Freud maintained that most morbid jealousy arose from suppressed homosexuality, and in some cases there is evidence to support this idea.

Morbid jealousy is a potentially dangerous condition and constitutes a powerful motive for homicide or serious assaults. The management depends on the associated psychiatric disorder. Where it is part of an affective disorder it is likely that it will respond to adequate treatment of the depression. In cases of schizophrenia the delusion may remit

---

* Quotation from *Morbid Jealousy and Murder* (R R Mowat) by courtesy of Tavistock Publications Ltd., London.

with appropriate treatment, or at least lose the affective drive. When secondary to alcoholism the condition may improve if the patient can be cured of his addiction. Where the delusions are not associated with evidence of other psychiatric illness they may respond to psychotherapy, but it is often necessary to arrange for at least a temporary separation of the partners if tragedy is to be avoided.

References

Schizophrenia

1   Schneider, K (1959) *Clinical Psychopathology*. Greve and Stratton, New York

Morbid Jealousy

2   Jaspers, K (1910) Eifersuchtwahn. *Zeitschrift für diagnostische Neurologie*, **1**, 367
3   Todd, J and Dewhurst, K (1967) *The Othello Syndrome in Some Uncommon Psychiatric Syndromes*. John Wright, Bristol
4   Mowat, R R (1966) *Morbid Jealousy and Murder*. Tavistock Publications, London

Further reading

Langfeldt, G (1961) The erotic jealousy syndrome. *Acta psychiatrica Scandinavica* (Suppl) **151**, 36
Shepherd, M (1961) Morbid jealousy: some clinical and social aspects of a psychiatric symptom. *Journal of Mental Science*, **107**, 687–753
Cobb, J (1979) Morbid jealousy. *British Journal of Hospital Medicine*, **21**, 5, 511

12. Cerebral Disease

Degenerative disorders of old age

The organic psychoses of old age are the commonest forms of cerebral disease presenting at out-patient clinics, and account for the vast majority of psychiatric hospital beds occupied by old people. With the increased number of aged people in the population, the prevalence of these conditions has also increased.

Old people are responsible for only a tiny part of the criminal offences that lead to conviction. Violent offences are very rare in the over-sixty group, and when they occur they are often associated with suicide attempts on the part of the offender. A small number are due to old men with paranoid disorders, or advanced chronic alcoholism. There is a relatively higher rate of sexual offences, the majority of which are committed by first offenders.

Old women commit very little crime and most of that is accounted for by theft, mainly in the form of shoplifting. Shoplifting by old men is mostly done by men with long histories of previous convictions who seem to have finally adopted this form of crime as their ability to perform more demanding criminal acts has declined.

In contrast, the majority of male sexual offenders are first offenders. The offences most often relate to indecent acts with children. These offences are often considered to be due to disinhibition caused by cerebral degeneration. In some cases, however, there is little evidence of intellectual impairment and the offender's behaviour in other respects appears to be normal. Many such offenders have suffered from life-long sexual difficulties. Their chances of establishing satisfactory sexual relationships with adults are extremely poor, and they may select children as their sexual object because of the relative ease with which a relationship can be established. While the relationship between sexual offences and early dementia may not always be clear or demonstrable, all elderly men charged with such offences should be fully psychiatrically investigated.

Violence in old age is most often directed at the self, and suicide reaches a peak incidence in late middle and old age. There is also a tendency to commit suicide by more violent means than those employed by young people. There is a link between suicide and cerebral degeneration, some 10% to 20% of elderly suicides having marked degenerative brain changes at post mortem [1].

Suicidal acts and attempted suicide by old people may be of forensic importance in that they may involve homicidal attacks on near relatives. Rarely such attacks occur without any associated suicidal ideas and may be provoked by quite trivial acts on the part of the victim. Such attacks may be carried out by old people who show little or no evidence of intellectual deterioration, but in whom there is evidence of blunting of affect and other personality changes.

Both suicide and homicide attempts may be made during confusional episodes in which there may be marked fluctuations both in level of consciousness and mood state. Such events can give rise to considerable diagnostic problems, as by the time the perpetrator is examined, the confusional state may have cleared. The examination and investigation of such cases is discussed later.

Presenile dementia

Obviously much that has been said about cerebral degeneration in the elderly applies equally to patients with dementing disorders developing before the senium. However, there are certain differences. First, the diagnosis may not be suspected in a younger person unless there is a clear family history of the illness which alerts concern. Secondly, the illness develops in a person who is, in other respects, still fit and healthy and thus capable of a wider range of criminal activities. Thirdly, the social and family environment is different. There is a likelihood that young children will still be living with the sufferer, providing potential victims for physical or sexual assault. The sufferer is most likely to be involved with men of his own age who may themselves be involved in criminal activities, and finally, alcohol is more likely to contribute to a loss of control and subsequent criminality.

Huntington's chorea has a particularly bad reputation of being associated with criminality. It has been claimed that non-affected sibs show a higher than normal incidence of such behaviour. The facts are less certain. Bolt [2] studied cases in the West of Scotland and came to the conclusion that crime was uncommon and that the majority of charges were trivial, though they included one case of infanticide. A study of cases by Dewhurst et al [3] showed that 18% had one or more convictions and a substantial number were admitted to hospital as a result of violence or abnormal sexual behaviour. This abnormal sexual behaviour included cases of morbid jealousy, indecent exposure, homosexual assault, incestuous sodomy, voyeurism and assault on females.

Oliver [4] also studied mental and social disorders of siblings not affected with the disease. He found a surprisingly high rate of childhood deaths, some of which were due to neglect or ill-treatment. In view of this treatment, it would be surprising if non-affected sibs did not show a higher than average incidence of disordered behaviour.

Traumatic brain damage

The acute effect of closed head injury is usually a change in the level of consciousness which may vary from a brief episode of confusion to prolonged coma or death. Such impairment may also occur with penetrating injuries or in those in which the static head is subjected to crushing pressures.

The length of time that unconsciousness persists is some indication as to the likelihood of permanent brain damage. As the level of unconsciousness lightens, the sufferer passes through a phase of disorientation usually proportional to the length of time of unconsciousness. In some cases this period of confusion leads into the stage of permanent dementia. During the period of confusion statements concerning the events leading up to the injury may be made by the patient which are not in fact true. This may be of medicolegal importance.

Amnesia

When consciousness is regained the patient may still not be able to record new information. Events preceding the injury may also be impossible to recall. Thus there may be both post-traumatic and retrograde amnesia.

The length of post-traumatic amnesia is defined as the time from the occurrence of the injury to the time when normal continuous memory was resumed. In some cases the point is rather vague, but in the majority the return of normal memory is abrupt.

The duration of retrograde amnesia is the time from the moment of injury to that of the last clear memory the patient can recall. The time is usually much shorter than for post-traumatic amnesia, though long periods of retrograde amnesia can occur after severe head injury. The duration of retrograde amnesia generally diminishes as recovery continues until only a few seconds or minutes cannot be recalled.

The duration of post-traumatic amnesia is a useful indication of the severity of the closed head injury, and correlates to some extent with prognosis. Thus it has been shown that patients with a post-traumatic amnesia of less than an hour are usually back at work within a month, while those with a post-traumatic amnesia longer than a week are unlikely to resume work in under a year.

Chronic states following head injury

Head injuries are responsible for a great deal of chronic disability. These disabilities include focal neurological defects and a variety of mental defects. The mental state reflects not only the specific neurological damage but the interplay between the organic factors and the premorbid personality and life situation of the sufferer. From the criminological point of view most interest centres round those cases in which personality changes occur with resultant criminality. Personality change following head injury may be very hard to evaluate. Many of the changes are exaggerations of personality traits which existed before the injury, but some, particularly in cases of frontal lobe damage, may be new. Changes in personality may be part of the global dementia or may occur in the presence of well preserved intellectual function.

In cases with intellectual impairment the personality changes are usually slowness, loss of drive and loss of interest. The emotions may be blunted or labile. The sufferer is often unstable and tends to be explosive if annoyed. Some become excessively passive and dependent and can be demanding and totally selfish.

People who have sustained frontal lobe damage may become tactless, feckless, facile and lacking in judgement and foresight. Inhibitions may be lost and sexual behaviour of an unacceptable nature indulged in. The severity of change may vary from an almost undetectable coarsening to a grossly disabling loss of control.

An aspect of personality change of particular legal importance is the loss of control of aggression. This change may occur in relative isolation and may be due to a relatively circumscribed lesion. The sufferer is liable to respond to quite trivial provocation with explosive outbursts of violence. Hooper (1945) [5] described such cases. These seem to differ from the generally irritable cases in that between episodes the sufferer seemed quite normal. In some it would seem to be an epileptic phenomenon, and E.E.G. studies may show a focal temporal lobe disturbance, in others it is related to the additional factor of alcohol intake.

Assessment

The diagnosis of dementia is an act of clinical judgement. Investigations may provide supporting evidence, but at present they cannot of themselves prove or disprove the diagnosis.

It is usual to employ some form of quantitative psychometric testing. Such tests include those which aim to provide some overall measure of intellectual function and those which set out to quantify specific aspects of memory or learning capacity.

The rationale of such tests is that certain intellectual abilities are less vulnerable to the effects of age and ageing (or of other forms of brain injury) than others. Weschler described this difference in relation to some of the sub-tests in his intelligence scale. He called those tests which were vulnerable 'Don't Hold' and those which were not affected 'Hold'. He suggested that by comparing a patient's scores on these sub-tests it would be possible to indicate the extent to which the patient's present intellectual capacity has deteriorated.

The use of these and other similar tests gives unreliable results and there is poor correlation between test scores and pathological and clinical findings.

Because of these difficulties, it is tempting to use specific tests which set out to measure the patient's present level of function and to compare his results with those of a sample population matched for age. Unfortunately much of the normative data is inadequate, failing to take account of different premorbid intellectual levels and individual differences for particular skills.

The most accurate results are those based on testing and then re-testing some months later. However, if the dementia is not due to a progressive lesion no change may be demonstrated, and in any event the clinician (and the lawyer) is interested in making a diagnosis now, not at some time in the future.

Wood (1979) [6] demonstrated the inadequacy of the WAIS* in diagnosing organic intellectual impairment when he found that in a

* Weschler Adult Intelligence Scale

series of patients shown to have large cerebral tumours by CAT scan the WAIS prediction was correct in only 22% of cases.

At present, the best way of assessing a patient with suspected dementia is to carry out a range of tests designed to demonstrate qualitatively a number of neuropsychological and cognitive processes which are known to be affected by organic disease, but not by emotional disorders.

Special investigations

Electroencephalogram (EEG)

At present conventional EEG studies do not show changes in cases of dementia consistent enough to provide a reliable diagnosis. Although localised slow waves in the EEG are sometimes indicative of focal arterial disease, they are not seen in all cases of arteriosclerosis. Focal disturbances in the temporal and occipital regions which in young people would be regarded as abnormal are found in apparently normal old people. Recent investigations by O'Connor et al [7] using computerised EEG analysis suggest that such techniques can distinguish between senile dementia, arteriosclerotic dementia and affective states in old people, but much further work is needed before this becomes an accepted finding. Space occupying lesions show up on EEG's in a high proportion of cases, and are sometimes indicated in the absence of other specific findings.

In general positive findings are of value, but negative findings do not exclude the possibility of organic brain disease.

Skull X-ray

The principal psychiatric indication for a straight X-ray of the skull is possibility of a cerebral tumour. Such a growth may be revealed by bony erosion or thickening of the vault. Osteolytic lesions may indicate the presence of multiple myelomatosis or secondary carcinomatosis. Erosion of the posterior clinoid processes may recur as a result of raised intra-cranial pressure, and enlargement of the pituitary fossa may indicate a pituitary tumour. A calcified pineal gland may be seen and can indicate a shift of the midline structures. Some tumours may themselves contain areas of calcification as may the cysts of cysticercosis.

Computerised tomography

This is a safe and reliable investigation, but at present the demand for it is such that it can only be used in cases where there are strong grounds for suspecting an organic lesion. It is chiefly of value in detecting cerebral tumours in which the method shows few false positive results, and equally few false negatives.

Scanning can also detect the presence of infarcted areas depending on the time it is performed after the cerebrovascular accident. The usual pattern is one of negative findings in the first 48 hours, becoming positive between 2 and 7 days, then a further negative phase.

The value of scan results in cases of cerebral atrophy is less well established. In part this reflects the present lack of normative data, but is also due to the lack of clear correlation between the degree of cerebral shrinkage as demonstrated and the severity of the dementing process as shown by psychometry and clinical examination.

Hypoglycaemia and automatism

Hypoglycaemia arising in a known diabetic would be unlikely to be regarded as a defence on the grounds that the sufferer should be aware of the possibility of such an event occurring and should recognise the prodromal signs early enough to take action (Watmore v Jenkins 1962) [8].

In cases of spontaneous hypoglycaemia, there is likely to be a history of recurrent transient episodes of altered behaviour or changes in level of consciousness, but the sufferer may not be aware of the nature of these episodes and they may be misinterpreted by others as being due to the taking of drugs or alcohol. This can be especially difficult as in some cases the taking of relatively modest amounts of alcohol can provoke the hypoglycaemia. The possibility that this condition is occurring should be borne in mind, and attention paid in taking the history to such features as transient episodes of confusion, slurring of speech, inappropriate instability, tremor and sweating and the like. If such episodes are reported by the individual or by relatives, an attempt should be made to establish the pattern of such attacks in relation to the time of day, meals, and exercise, as this may give clues as to the underlying mechanism. Enquiry should also be made into the diet, bowel habits, drinking habits and past medical history with special reference to treatment for gastric ulceration or surgical operations on the gut.

Having established the possibility of spontaneous hypoglycaemia the appropriate physical investigations must be performed.

Hypoglycaemia is defined as a blood glucose level below 49 mg/100 ml (3 mmol/l). Symptoms may develop at higher values than this if there has been a rapid fall from a previously high level. Some people do not show symptoms even at 30 mg/100 ml (1.8 mmol/l).

Causes

1. Insulin or drug induced hypoglycaemia
While insulin induced hypoglycaemia is common in diabetics it has been used in suicide attempts, and theoretically could be used as a means of homicide. Sulphonylureas may induce hypoglycaemia.

2. Hyperinsulinism
A rare cause of spontaneous hypoglycaemia is an insulin secreting tumour of the pancreas. The tumour is usually benign and may be single or multiple. Attacks of hypoglycaemia generally occur at night or just before breakfast. Personality and behavioural changes may be the first feature.

3. Hypoglycaemia may occur in adrenal or pituitary insufficiency.

4. Non pancreatic tumours
Certain malignant tumours can cause spontaneous hypoglycaemia. It is most commonly associated with retroperitoneal tumours of mesodermal origin. The mechanism is not known.

5. Reactive hypoglycaemia
Certain food substances can trigger off hypoglycaemia in some individuals. These sensitivity reactions mostly occur in young children.

6. Functional reactive hypoglycaemia
Some people develop hypoglycaemia 2 to 4 hours after a meal. This is an exaggeration of the normal dip below the fasting level which occurs after some 2 to 3 hours. A similar reaction may be seen in patients following a gastrectomy; typically such patients have a 'lag' storage glucose tolerance curve. In some early cases of diabetes hypoglycaemia is seen 3 to 5 hours after the intake of carbohydrates.

7. Alcohol-induced hypoglycaemia
Hypoglycaemia may develop 2 to 10 hours after drinking alcohol—

usually in substantial amounts. It may only be demonstrated if the patient fasts for up to 72 hours before being given alcohol.

Diagnosis

(a)   Seventy-two-hour fast
Random or even fasting blood sugar levels may fail to demonstrate hypoglycaemia. It is necessary to fast for 72 hours to disprove the existence of spontaneous hypoglycaemia. Normal subjects and those with reactive hypoglycaemia will not develop a low blood glucose level under those conditions. Failure to develop hypoglycaemia after fasting for 72 hours almost disproves the presence of an insuloma. The test should only be carried out in hospital with constant observation.

(b)   Prolonged glucose tolerance test
A normal glucose tolerance test is carried out with samples of blood taken at 30-minute intervals for 5 or 6 hours instead of the usual 3 hours. This test is only of value in demonstrating reactive functional hypoglycaemia.

(c)   Alcohol-induced
After fasting for 12 to 72 hours, a blood sugar level is taken and the patient given 50 to 60 ml of alcohol. Blood samples are taken for glucose estimation at half-hourly intervals.

The demonstration of spontaneous or reactive hypoglycaemia is merely the first step in establishing the defence, for it must be shown that such falls in blood sugar are associated with changes in the level of consciousness. Careful observations must be made and recorded throughout the tests and the findings correlated with the blood glucose levels.

The tests should be performed while the patient's EEG is recorded and blood levels, behavioural changes and EEG findings should be correlated. Finally, the conditions preceding the events leading to the change should be reduplicated as accurately as possible and a similar monitory of the blood levels and EEG and behavioural changes recorded.

To summarise—it is necessary to demonstrate:

(1)   That the offender is liable to develop hypoglycaemia under certain defined conditions.
(2)   Then during such an episode his behaviour or level of consciousness changes.

(3) That at the time of the offence it is likely that hypoglycaemia had been provoked.

References

Cerebral disease

1 Sainsbury, P (1962) Suicide in later life. *Gerontologia clinica*, **4**, 161
2 Bolt, J M W (1970) Huntington's chorea in the west of Scotland. *British Journal of Psychiatry*, **116**, 259–270
3 Dewhurst, K, Oliver, J E and McKnight, A L (1970) Socio-psychiatric consequences of Huntington's disease. *British Journal of Psychiatry*, **116**, 255–258
4 Oliver, J E (1970) Huntington's chorea in Northamptonshire. *British Journal of Psychiatry*, **116**, 241–253

Traumatic brain damage

5 Hooper, R S, McGregor, J M and Nathan, P W (1945) Explosive rage following head injuries. *Journal of Mental Science*, **91**, 458–471
6 Wood, R Llewellyn (1980) The relationship of brain damage measured by computerised axial tomography to quantitative intellect impairment. Research in *Psychology & Medicine, vol 1* (Ed Grimeberg, Oborne, Elsen) Academic Press, London
7 Shaw, J C, O'Connor, K P and Ongley, C (1977) Investigation. *British Journal of Psychiatry*, **130**, 260–264

Hypoglycaemia and automatism

8 Watmore *v* Jenkins (1962) 2 Q.B. 572

Further reading

Hill, D, Sargant, W and Heppenstall, M (1943) *Lancet*, **i**, 526–527
Bovill, D (1973) A case of functional hypoglycaemia. *British Journal of Psychiatry*, **123**, 353–358

13. Epilepsy

People who suffer from epilepsy have historically been treated with a curious mixture of fear, suspicion and reverence. Known to the Greeks as the 'falling sickness' or the 'sacred disease' it provoked Hippocrates [1] to write, 'it appears to me to be no wise more divine nor more sacred than other diseases, but has a natural cause from which it originates like other affections'. In 1889 Lombroso, an Italian criminologist implied in his book 'L'Uomo Delinquente' that all crime had an epileptic basis, though he was using epileptic in a much more diffuse way than its present meaning [2]. However, by the 1920s the pendulum was beginning to swing in the opposite direction. W. C. Sullivan [3], who was Medical Superintendent of Broadmoor, showed that the proportion of epileptics among the patients admitted to Broadmoor averaged about 7% of males and 5% of females, which were almost identical to the figures for patients admitted to non-criminal lunatic asylums.

In 1950 Alstrom [4] studied patients attending a neurological clinic in Sweden and concluded that the prevalence of criminal behaviour in the epileptics was the same as in the general population. The study, however, excludes those epileptics who for some reason were confined to institutions.

In 1966, Gudmundsson [5] published a survey of all the epileptics in Iceland that could be traced. This study showed that the number of male epileptics convicted of criminal offences was three times that of the general population. However, many of these offences were for breaches of liquor laws and customs and control regulations.

In 1952 Hill and Pond [6] investigated 105 cases of murder, and found nine cases with specific EEG changes, and nine cases with a clear history of epileptic seizures but a normal EEG. A similar study by Driver et al [7] in 1974, however, showed an incidence of EEG abnormalities of 10%.

In 1969 Gunn [8] reported a survey of epileptics in British prisons which showed an incidence of 7/8 per 1,000 which is significantly higher than the figures found in surveys of the general population.

While it is not possible on present evidence to be sure whether or not the incidence of criminality is higher amongst epileptics, it would seem that being epileptic carries a greater risk of being institutionalised.

One of the difficulties in carrying out research on epilepsy is the difficulty in arriving at a definition of the disorder which is operationally reliable, practical and generally acceptable to other workers in the field.

A comprehensive attempt at definition is that of Gastaut et al [9] which includes clinical, EEG, anatomical and aetiological factors. For epidemiological studies, however, a much more simple definition has to suffice. A number of such studies have been carried out, though they are not strictly comparable because of differences in definition and methodology. The rate per 100 of the population varied from 0.6 to 6.2 but the lowest figures were in surveys of a highly selected student population. In the UK the figure usually quoted by the British Epilepsy Association of 5 in 1000 would seem to be reasonably accurate.

The College of General Practitioners [10] carried out a prevalence study in 1960 using as their definition 'attacks primarily cerebral in origin, in which there is disturbance of movement, feeling, behaviour or consciousness, excluding fainting, aural vertigo and psychologically determined attacks'. This was a purely clinical definition, taking no account of EEG findings.

It is not possible at present to be certain what factors lead to the greater incidence of epilepsy found in prisoners, but one or more of the following factors may play a part:

(1) The underlying brain disorder leads not only to epileptic attacks, but to criminal behaviour as well.

(2) The underlying brain disorder is itself a result of experiences which themselves predispose to later criminality, e.g. battering as a child.

(3) Personality factors leading to behaviour which results in both anti-social and self damaging acts, the latter including brain damage and subsequent epilepsy.

(4) Being epileptic produces social and inter-personal difficulties which in turn may lead to anti-social acts. Epileptics may have difficulty in obtaining employment and be debarred from certain occupations.

As far as the individual offender is concerned, the relationship of his epilepsy and the crime can be considered under the following headings:

(a)   Did he commit the offence during an epileptic seizure?

(b)   Did he commit the offence during a postictal confusional state?

(c)   Though not directly related to the offence, is his epilepsy symptomatic of an underlying brain disorder which itself is relevant to the offence?

(d)   If the crime is not causally linked to the epilepsy or the underlying brain disorder, to what extent should the disorder be taken into account in determining the appropriate sentence?

Offences committed during the seizure

In cases where the seizure involves rapid loss of consciousness followed by involuntary muscle movements, the ability to commit an offence is obviously quite limited apart from the situation where the offender is driving a motor vehicle. It is in cases where the seizure causes behavioural automatism that the possibility of criminal offences being committed arises.

The prevalence of epileptic automatism is difficult to estimate and depends on the population studies. A study by Margerison (1961) [11] of patients in an epileptic colony found that almost a third of the patients had episodes of automatic behaviour. However, a study of epileptic patients attending an out-patient department (Knox 1968) [12] reported that only 10% had a history of automatism. This difference may be accounted for by the fact that patients who are institutionalised for their epilepsy are much more likely to be suffering from temporal lobe epilepsy and it is this form which is most likely to produce automatic behaviour. Automatism as a manifestation of seizure activity rarely occurs as the sole manifestation of the epilepsy; in most patients it occurs in combination with other seizure patterns, notably with grand mal attacks.

In cases of temporal lobe automatism the patient may first experience an aura, most commonly consisting of abdominal sensations.

The behaviour during an attack is very variable both between patients and in the same patient at different times. The fact that the behaviour is automatic may not be noticed by people unfamiliar with the patient as the activity may seem purposeful and well executed. In general, the sequence of events is an initial suspension of activity, followed by repetitive stereotyped activity, and finally complex semi-purposeful behaviour which merges into normality. During the period of automatism, the patient may continue to perform quite complex activities, but even so his judgement and awareness are impaired. Most periods of automatic behaviour are short-lasting, up to five minutes, a few last up to fifteen minutes and no observed case has lasted for more than an hour (Knox 1968) [12]. Amnesia for the episode is complete in the majority of cases, but anterograde amnesia is not found. Violence appears to be rare during automatism and when it occurs is mostly due to attempts to interfere with the automatic behaviour of the sufferer.

Postictal confusional states

It is obviously impossible to distinguish retrospectively whether a particular act was committed as part of a psychomotor seizure or during a brief period of confusion following the cessation of the actual seizure. However, in some cases of grand mal epilepsy and in cases of petit mal epilepsy there is clear evidence of a confusional state persisting for some time after the seizures have ended. It is rare for serious violence to occur during such episodes.

In order to assess the likelihood that a crime has been committed during a period of epileptic automatism, the following factors should be considered:

(1) There should be a past history of definite epileptic attacks, preferably including forms of seizures other than episodes of automatic behaviour.

(2) Automatism does not have to have occurred previously and it certainly need not be a regular feature of previous seizures.

(3) The diagnosis must be based on clinical evidence. An abnormal EEG does not establish a diagnosis, though it lends support. A negative EEG proves nothing.

(4) The onset of the allegedly automatic behaviour should be abrupt, and it should persist for only a relatively brief time.

(5) The behaviour should be relatively inappropriate and there should be no evidence of premeditation and planning.

(6) The subject should be amnesic for the event but there should not be anterograde amnesia.

(7) Observers may have noted some signs of impaired awareness such as failure to reply appropriately to questions, a dazed or vacant expression, meaningless verbal statements or confused

wandering. However, untrained observers may fail to notice anything peculiar about the defendant's behaviour.

The differential diagnosis includes:

(a) Hysterical fugue states
(b) Malingering
(c) Other causes of confusional states
(d) Somnambulism.

Investigation

(1) Full EEG studies including sleep recordings should be performed. Sphenoidal lead recordings may help in cases of temporal lobe epilepsy.
(2) Straight skull X-ray may be helpful.
(3) EMI scan studies have now largely replaced air encephalography and arteriograms.
(4) Psychometric assessment may help to demonstrate frontal lobe damage, or help to lateralise temporal lobe lesions.

References

Epilepsy

1   Hippocrates. *On the Sacred Disease:* Hippocratic Writings. Encyclopaedia Britannica, Chicago
2   Lombroso, C (1889) *L'Uomo Delinquente*. Bocca, Turin
3   Sullivan, W C (1924) *Crime and Insanity*. Arnold, London
4   Alstrom, C H (1950) Epilepsy. *Acta psychiatrica et neurologica Scandinavica*, Suppl. 63, p. 394
5   Gudmundsson, G (1966) Epilepsy in Iceland. *Acta neurologica Scandinavica*, **43**, Suppl. 25
6   Hill, D and Pond, D A (1952) Reflections on 100 capital cases submitted to EEG. *Journal of Mental Science*, **98**, 23–43
7   Driver, M U, West, L R and Faulk, M (1974) Clinical and EEG studies of prisoners charged with murder. *British Journal of Psychiatry*, **125**, 583–587
8   Gunn, J and Fenton, G W (1969) Epilepsy in prisons. *British Medical Journal*, **4**, 326–329
9   Gastaut, H et al (1964) A proposed international classification of epileptic seizures. *Epilepsia*, **5**, 297–306

10 College of General Practitioners (1960) *British Medical Journal*, **2**, 416–422

11 Margerison, J H and Corsells, J A N (1961) *Brain*, **89**, 499

12 Knox, (1968) Epileptic automatism and violence. *Medicine, Science and the Law*, **8**, 96–104

Further reading

Fenton, G W (1972) Epilepsy and automatism. *British Journal of Hospital Medicine*, **7**, 57–64

Gunn, J (1977) *Epileptics in Prison*. Academic Press, London

Gunn, J and Fenton, G W (1971) Epilepsy, automatism and crime. *Lancet*, **i**, 1173–1176

Kligman, D and Goldberg, D A (1975) Temporal lobe epilepsy and aggression. *Journal of Nervous and Mental Diseases*, **160**, 324–341

14. Subnormality and Chromosome Abnormalities

Subnormality

The 1959 Mental Health Act defined subnormality as 'A state of incomplete development of mind (not amounting to severe subnormality) which includes subnormality of intelligence and which requires or is susceptible to medical treatment or other special care or training of the patient'.

Severe subnormality was defined as 'a state of arrested or incomplete development of mind which includes subnormality of intelligence and is of such a nature or degree that the patient is incapable of living an independent life or of guarding himself against serious exploitation or will be so incapable when of an age to do so'.

The above definitions contain social, psychological and medical components and it is difficult to know what weight should be given to each of them in the practical situation. The 1959 Act avoids setting quantifiable limits to what is or is not to be regarded as subnormality of intelligence.

The notion of 'intelligence' is relatively recent; previously it was dealt with by psychologists under such headings as reason, intellect, and judgement. Interest in the concept of intelligence and its measurement began with the publication of 'Le développement de l'intelligence chez les enfants' by A. Binet in 1908. Most of the subsequent work has been directed at identifying the basic factors of 'intelligence'. It is important to remember, however, that general intelligence is not synonymous with intellectual ability, and it cannot be treated in isolation, but must be considered in the general setting of the individual's personality structure.

Intelligence can be defined as the 'global capacity of the individual to act purposefully, to think rationally and to deal effectively with his environment'. All measures of 'intelligence' actually consist of tests of specific types of performance, combined into a collection of tests which give some indication of the individual's overall ability.

Intelligence as measured seems to be due in part to innate ability and in part to environmental factors such as education, intellectual stimulation and emotional state. The innate ability is transmitted polygenetically and, like other inherited features involving large numbers of genes, its distribution within a population follows a 'normal' curve. The majority of people who have below average intelligence do not have any specific brain disease to account for it, any more than most short people have any disease causing their lack of height. There are, however, numerous conditions which interfere with brain development and may thus lead to low intelligence in the sufferer. Almost all cases of severe subnormality are due to pathological processes and are often accompanied by a variety of physical handicaps as well.

A convenient way of expressing an individual's level of intelligence is that known as IQ (intelligence quotient). This is arrived at by dividing the subject's mental age (MA) by his chronological age (CA) and multiplying by 100. The mental age is arrived at by matching the subject's score on standard tests to the average score for a particular age group.

An individual's IQ is relatively constant for those of average intelligence, but is less so for individuals well above or well below average. The concept of IQ has been much criticised and of itself is of limited value; however, it provides a convenient method of comparing individuals with their peers. In very general terms people whose IQ score is below 50 fall into the severely subnormal category, those between 50 and 70 into the subnormal category, while those between 70 and 80 are likely to have educational difficulties and require special help. Such measures of intelligence, however, should only form a part of the assessment, attention being paid, when determining appropriate management, to the degree of social inadequacy or incompetence.

Low or limited intelligence may make life in ordinary society more than usually difficult. In some ways those with less severe handicap are placed under greater stress, as less allowance is made for their intellectual difficulties which indeed may not be recognised. Such stress may lead to the development of psychiatric disorders in addition to the intellectual difficulties already present.

For many years it was believed that the criminal population was less intelligent than the law abiding but this was due to errors in the research, reflecting social and cultural differences rather than differences in innate intelligence.

More recent surveys have shown that only about 3% of delinquent youths had IQ's falling in the subnormal range. The majority of offenders with low IQ's are derived from those whose intellectual handicap reflects normal variation rather than those with specific syndromes. This in part may be due to the fact that many such syndromes impose more or less severe physical handicaps on the sufferer as well as limited intelligence. There is also a high correlation between limited intelligence and social deprivation in those who offend.

The only close association between low IQ and criminal behaviour which has survived more sophisticated research is that with sexual offences, subnormal male offenders being committed for sexual crimes six times more frequently than other offenders [1]. The commonest sexual offence is indecent exposure. Indecent assaults by subnormal men are often carried out on victims who know the offender and thus carry a high detection rate. Assaults on young children may reflect the difficulty the adult subnormal has in establishing relationships with women of his own age.

Arson may be committed by subnormals as a result of a childish desire for excitement, or as a method of gaining revenge on someone in authority. Occasionally, it may be used as 'a cry for help'.

Subnormals also form part of what has aptly been described as the 'stage army' of offender-patients who drift between prison and hospital, and tend to gravitate to large cities where they swell the numbers of the homeless.

Examination of the mentally handicapped offenders

Examination may be difficult because of the defendant's limited powers of comprehension and expression. The first task is usually to assess the offender's fitness to plead. The majority of subnormals and borderline cases are fit to plead in the absence of other factors such as superadded psychotic illness. The defending Counsel may need to spend much more time with the offender explaining in simple language the nature of the charge and the difference between a guilty and non-guilty plea. In fact time is of the essence in examining such a client. The subnormal's replies to questions are likely to be monosyllabic and thus not lead on to any further discussion of the situation. The examiner is likely to exhaust his store of stock questions very quickly and find that he is little wiser than when he started.

The interview may need to be supplemented by information from relatives, school teachers and social workers. Special examinations may be of great help. Proper psychological testing not only establishes a base line IQ, but can also demonstrate the presence of specific learning difficulties which may require, or be susceptible to, special methods of training.

Physical examination should be done to determine the nature of any associated physical handicaps and where relevant EEG's and chromosome studies should be performed.

The placement of mentally handicapped offenders frequently presents a problem. The seriousness of the offence and the 'dangerousness' of the offenders are often such as not to justify the maximum security provisions of the Special Hospitals. Most areas of the country still do not have hospitals offering medium secure units. The fully 'open' hospital may well reject the offender as being more than can be coped with in an open setting. This is particularly true of sex offenders and arsonists.

Chromosome abnormalities

Tjio and Levan [2] established in 1956 that the normal chromosome number in man is 46. The sex chromosomes are known as X and Y. A normal female has two X chromosomes and a normal male has one X and one Y. In general if a Y chromosome is present the individual develops as a male irrespective of the number of X chromosomes present. In the absence of a Y chromosome the individual develops as a female.

In 1949 Barr and Bertram [3] described a dark staining mass of chromatin in the nuclei of non-dividing female cells which was not present in male cells. Female cells were, therefore, said to be chromatin positive. In 1942 Klinefelter [4] described a syndrome in which males who, having appeared physically normal up to the age of puberty, were found to have testicular atrophy. Some had evidence of feminisation and mental subnormality was found in some cases. Later it was found that patients with this condition had an additional X chromosome (47 XXY). Similar physical findings exist in men with two additional X chromosomes (48 XXXY) and also in males with 48 XXYY chromosomes. The latter are in general taller than the others.

The incidence of abnormal chromosome counts in the public at large is not known with absolute certainty but are said to be: [5]

1 in 2,000 of extra Y chromosomes in adult males
1 in 500 of extra X chromosomes in adult males.

The frequency of chromosome abnormalities in males in hospitals for the mentally handicapped has been found to be higher by a factor of five or six than in the general population [6].

The role of chromosome abnormalities in determining abnormal behaviour remains unclear. It has been found in special hospitals which select their population on the basis of a combination of subnormality and serious anti-social behaviour that the incidence of chromosome abnormalities (particularly 48 XXYY) was higher than in ordinary subnormality hospitals [7]. When the total male population of Carstairs Special Hospital was screened for chromosome abnormalities it was found that those males with a 47 XYY complement were on average 10.5 cm taller than the patients with normal chromosomes. The XYY group also differed in their criminal history in that they got into trouble at an earlier age, their crimes were mostly against property, and there was less family history of criminal activity [8]. However, when an unselected population of young delinquents was studied [9] the incidence of chromosome abnormalities did not differ significantly from the incidence in the general population.

It is possible that it is not the chromosome abnormality that is directly responsible for the anti-social behaviour but the combination of low IQ and great size, which not only leads to disturbed behaviour, but provokes a penal sentence from the Court and thus accounts for the disproportionate numbers of such people in the Special Hospitals.

Legal aspects

The presence or absence of chromosome abnormalities does not of itself affect criminal liability. The presence of such an abnormality might be used to support the diagnosis of subnormality. It might also be used as part of an argument that a hospital order would be the most appropriate form of disposal.

(Note: In this chapter, the term subnormality has been used in preference to the phrase mental handicap, as subnormality is at present used in legal texts, and in the 1959 Mental Health Act.)

References

Subnormality and chromosome abnormalities

Subnormality

1 Power, D J (1969) Subnormality and crime I. *Medicine, Science and the Law*, **9**, 83–93; and

Power, D J (1969) Subnormality and crime II. *Medicine, Science and the Law,* **9,** 162–171

Further reading

James, F E and Snaith, R P (Eds) (1979) *Psychiatric Illness and Mental Handicap.* Gaskell Press, London

Chromosome abnormalities
2   Tjio, J H and Levan, A (1956) The chromosome number of man. *Hereditas (Lund),* **42,** 1
3   Barr, M L and Bertram, E G (1949) A morphological distinction between necromes of the male and female. *Nature (London),* **163,** 676
4   Klinefelter, H F et al (1942) Syndrome characterised by gynaecomastia, etc. *Journal of Clinical Endocrinology,* **2,** 615
5   McLean, N, Hardner, D G and Court Brown, W M (1961) Abnormalities of sex chromosome constitution in newborn babies. *Lancet,* **ii,** 406
6   Ferguson Smith, M A (1958) Chromatin positive Klinefelter's syndrome in a mental deficiency hospital. *Lancet,* **i,** 1327
7   Casey, M D et al (1966) Sex chromosome abnormalities in two state hospitals. *Nature (London),* **209,** 641
8   Price, W H and Whatmore, P B (1967) Behaviour disorders and patterns of crime among XYY males identified at a maximum security hospital. *British Medical Journal,* **1,** 533
9   Court Brown, W M (1968) Cytogenic studies in humans. *Proceedings of the Royal Society of Medicine,* **61,** 164

15. Alcohol and Drug Abuse

Alcohol

The relationship between criminal acts and alcohol can be considered under two broad headings. First, crimes committed by those who are intoxicated at the time, and secondly, crimes committed by people suffering from disorders resulting from excessive alcohol intake over a protracted period.

Immediate effects

The major effect of alcohol is on the brain and these effects are related to the dosage. At blood levels of 50 mg% the person experiences a lifting of normal inhibitions and a diminution in anxiety. Motor skills become affected at levels over 30 mg% and are seriously impaired at over 80 mg%. The majority of people are severely intoxicated at concentrations of 300 mg% and at levels above this confusion, stupor and death may occur. The fatal concentration usually lies between 500 mg% and 800 mg%.

The higher the level of blood alcohol the greater the impairment of the powers of judgement. The person is, therefore, less able to recognise how impaired his performance has become and is thus more likely to take risks.

The effects of alcohol on mood are complex and are much influenced by the setting in which the drinking is done. In convivial company the effect is usually to increase contentment, cheerfulness and euphoria. However, such moods can be rapidly changed to lachrymose unhappiness or unbridled aggression by quite trivial events.

The general disinhibition may allow of overt sexual behaviour or invitations to such behaviour in individuals who are normally over-shy, lacking in confidence, or guilt ridden. This liberation of sexual drive by alcohol may be accompanied by a loss of ability to perform and the resulting failure may lead to aggressive episodes.

Drunkenness offences

Being drunk in a public place has been a criminal offence for more than three hundred years. In 1977 in England and Wales the Magistrates' Courts found 41,581 males (and 3,360 females) over the age of 21, guilty of simple drunkenness, while a further 33,842 males and 3,069 females were found guilty of aggravated drunkenness. Only six of these cases resulted in the making of a hospital order, the vast majority being fined.

A study of cases of drunkenness coming before Camberwell Magistrates' Court was reported by Howard et al [1]. They found that only a small number of such offenders saw their problems in terms of an illness and used medical or psychiatric facilities. The researchers felt that in the majority of cases the drinking was best considered as a learned behavioural response to a variety of personal and social pressures. They considered that such cases were best referred to those community agencies which attempt to relieve those pressures and teach new non-drinking modes of coping.

The other way in which alcohol may be the direct cause of a criminal act is in relationship to the laws concerning motor vehicles. This aspect has been discussed under Road Traffic Offences (chapter 9).

The chronic alcohol abuser may develop a number of physical and mental conditions which may be a factor in criminality and which may provide a defence against the charge, or may be taken in mitigation.

Alcoholic 'blackouts'

These are episodes of profound amnesia for events which have occurred in the course of a drinking bout. The events 'forgotten' may be of considerable significance and the length of amnesia is usually several hours but may cover days. The behaviour of the sufferer during the period of amnesia may appear to be relatively normal. Criminal acts or grossly abnormal forms of behaviour may occasionally occur during such episodes. In these cases the question of malingering has to be considered. The onset of amnesia is usually acute, and the return of normal memory is also usually abrupt. Such episodes are commoner amongst spirit drinkers than among imbibers of wine or beer. The occurrence of blackouts is closely related to the severity and duration of alcoholism. The most extensive studies of these conditions are those of Goodwin et al [2, 3]. They studied a randomly selected group of 100 hospitalised alcoholics and found that 64 had experienced memory loss in association with drinking. Their data suggested that there are two types of alcoholic blackout. One type has a definite beginning, ends with feeling of 'lost time' and is rarely followed by a return of memory. The second type is when the subject is unaware of the amnesic period until the events occurring during it are spontaneously recalled later, or the subject is told of the events by other people. In this type, eventual recall almost always occurs. Both sorts of blackouts were associated with extreme degrees of intoxication, yet during the episodes the person was fully conscious and capable of performing complicated and purposeful acts.

At present the mode of action of alcohol in producing these amnesic states is not clearly known.

Withdrawal symptoms

After a period of alcohol abuse the body appears to become adjusted to a certain level of circulating alcohol. When this level drops as a result of abstinence a variety of symptoms may develop. The exact mechanism of these disorders remains uncertain, though their severity seems to be linked to the amount of alcohol drunk and the length of time for which it has been taken.

The earliest signs and symptoms of the onset of withdrawal phenomena are usually tremulousness and nausea. Short lasting hallucinations may also occur. These signs may develop within 3 to 12 hours of stopping drinking. Some patients develop epileptiform seizures, usually between 12 to 48 hours after stopping drinking, though they may occur much later on. These fits do not imply an underlying epileptic predisposition. In about a third of cases the sufferer goes on to show the symptoms of delirium tremens.

Delirium tremens

This condition still carries a substantial risk of death. The full blown state consists of profound confusion, marked tremor and vivid hallucinations. The sufferer is restless and agitated. Such cases are relatively uncommon as compared to tremulousness, transient hallucinosis and fits. The onset is relatively abrupt and often occurs at night. The patient is restless and agitated and may seem very alert though, in fact, his awareness of his surroundings is impaired. He is confused and disorientated.

The hallucinations may be visual or auditory and are very vivid. The auditory hallucinations may be threatening or persecutory in nature. The visual hallucinations may be terrifying and often consist of small animals such as rats or snakes. Occasionally Lilliputian hallucinations occur in which small figures perform involved activities, such as battles or sporting contests. The hallucinations produce strong emotional responses from the sufferer, commonly of terror but sometimes of amusement. The disorder usually lasts for only a few days, often ending in a period of sleep. It is a serious medical emergency and must be treated energetically by sedation, fluid replacement and high potency vitamin injections. During an episode the sufferer may become aggressive or self destructive.

Alcoholic hallucinosis

Relatively rarely a condition of hallucinosis may develop in a setting of clear consciousness. Initially, the hallucinations are usually auditory and simple in nature, consisting of noises such as bangs, the noise of burning, or of water running. Gradually they take on the form of spoken words. These are generally derogatory or accusatory. They may consist of instructions to the sufferer, which can lead to some form of bizarre behaviour. The person may develop secondary delusions based on the hallucinations. This syndrome has to be distinguished from schizophrenia. The vast majority of such cases are short-lived, clearing completely within a few days or weeks and leaving no residual mental symptoms. About 20% go on to develop a chronic state, either resembling schizophrenia, or developing an amnesic state.

Drugs

According to the World Health Organisation (1969) 'Drugs refer to any substance which when taken into the living organism may modify one or more of its functions'.

People take drugs for one or more of the following reasons:

(1) To cure a disease
(2) To relieve symptoms of a disease
(3) To alter a normal mental state
    (a) to one of increased awareness
    (b) to one of diminished awareness
    (c) to one of abnormal awareness

(4) To remove an unpleasant mental state
(5) To induce a pleasant mental state.

The first two reasons are regarded as legitimate, the rest are tolerated within certain limits. When these limits are exceeded the person is said to be abusing the drug. Drug abuse is defined as 'persistent or sporadic excessive drug-use inconsistent with or unrelated to acceptable medical practice'. Drug abuse *per se* cannot be regarded as an illness, though it may be the symptom of an illness and may itself cause illness. Using drugs may lead to the development of a dependence which may be either psychological or physiological, or both. The World Health Organisation offers a definition:

'Drug dependence is a state, psychic and also sometimes physical, resulting from the interaction between a living organism and a drug, characterised by behavioural and other responses that always include a compulsion to take the drugs on a continuous or periodic basis in order to experience its psychic effects, and sometimes to avoid the discomfort of its absence. Tolerance may or may not be present. A person may be dependent on more than one drug.'

The types of drugs which may be abused include almost any substance which produces some change in the taker's mental state, but they can be classified into three main types (with a degree of overlap of action in some drugs):

(1) Drugs which have a mainly *sedative* action
(2) Drugs which have a mainly *stimulant* action
(3) Drugs which have an *hallucinogenic* action.

Sedative drugs

These may be considered under two headings:

(i) Narcotic analgesics—these have powerful pain relieving effects and also produce changes in consciousness, e.g. opiates.
(ii) Sedative drugs—used to produce sleep or daytime sedation, e.g. barbiturates and barbiturate-like sedatives; tranquillisers.

Alcohol has sedative properties but as it has almost no medical uses it is considered separately.

Narcotic analgesics
These drugs have a high level of dependency-producing potential. The

best known members of this group are morphine, diamorphine (heroin), physeptone (methadone) and pethidine.

The opiates and synthetic analgesics

The major effects of drugs of this type are pain relief, the diminution of anxiety, and euphoria. Repeated use of this type of drug produces both psychological and physical dependence. The user develops a strong craving for the drug and becomes extremely distressed when unable to obtain it. Gradually the drug takes over the life of the user so that he spends almost all his time thinking about the drug and ways of obtaining it. This encourages addicts to seek out the company of others equally preoccupied, and so develops a drug-taking sub-culture.

Physical dependence is demonstrated by the development of withdrawal symptoms when the drug is stopped. Mild symptoms include yawning, running eyes and nose, sweating and loss of appetite. More prolonged withdrawal leads to trembling, abdominal cramps and sleeplessness, while more severe symptoms of restlessness, vomiting, diarrhoea and weight loss may occur.

Apart from the direct physical consequences of taking the drug, there are the secondary risks involved in self-administered injections. Sterile precautions are rarely observed, so that the risk of local or generalised infection is high. The greatest risk comes from the using of shared needles with the transmission of viral hepatitis. Overdosage is also a risk, particularly after periods of enforced abstinence, when tolerance of the drug has diminished.

Barbiturates

Barbiturate dependency is a relatively common condition in middle-aged and elderly people. Barbiturate addiction is becoming increasingly common amongst young people who are tending to use them in place of or as well as opiate derivatives.

Acute intoxication is commonly seen either as a result of suicide attempts or due to accidental overdosage in addicts. There is usually a short period of confusion and drowsiness which is rapidly followed by increasing coma. In the early phase nystagmus may be a marked feature.

Dangers of barbiturates

Barbiturates, particularly by injection, are extremely dangerous in that there is a relatively small difference between the therapeutic and the lethal dosage. Tolerance develops fairly quickly and allows the addict to survive much greater doses than the normal. Tolerance is, however, lost rapidly if the drug is not used for a time, and this may lead to the addict giving himself a lethal dose by basing the amount used on his previous dose level. Barbiturates also potentiate the effects of alcohol and opiate drugs.

Chronic barbiturate intoxication

This produces a state very similar to alcoholic intoxication, with impaired awareness, slurred speech and unsteadiness of gait. When the drug is withdrawn there is at first some improvement, but after eight to twelve hours, withdrawal symptoms start to appear. The sufferer becomes anxious, tremulous, nauseated and dizzy. This may progress to vomiting and postural hypotension. After 48 to 72 hours, more severe symptoms may develop, including grand mal fits and delirium—closely resembling DTs, with auditory and visual hallucinations. The daily dose of barbiturates likely to produce physical dependence lies between 600 mg and 800 mg (pentobarbitone). The higher the daily dose, the greater the severity of the withdrawal symptoms. Differentiation between barbiturate and other forms of intoxication depends on estimations of serum barbiturate levels.

Stimulant drugs

Amphetamines

The most widely abused drugs in this group are the amphetamines and amphetamine-like substances. The effect of the drug varies from person to person, but the commonest effect is one of increased confidence, euphoria and alertness. This mood can easily change into one of increased irritability, argumentativeness and explosive violence. When the effects of the drug wear off, the user may experience periods of profound despondency and lethargy. These feelings may encourage further amphetamine taking. Many users also take barbiturates or barbiturate-like drugs to terminate the wakefulness produced by the amphetamines, so that multiple dependence is common.

Some chronic amphetamine abusers develop an amphetamine psychosis. This is a schizophrenic-like episode in which the sufferer may hear hallucinatory voices and develop ideas of persecution.

Tolerance to amphetamine develops rapidly. There seems to be no real physical dependence on the drug, but psychological dependence may be extreme.

The other important stimulant drug is cocaine.

Cocaine

Cocaine is a powerful stimulant of the central nervous system. Its use can produce states of excitement, elation and euphoria. It seems to produce little physical dependence, but rapidly leads to psychological dependence. It is taken either by sniffing it up the nostrils, where it is absorbed through the nasal mucosa, or by injecting into a vein, when it is often combined with heroin. When sniffed, it tends to ulcerate the nasal passages and may produce considerable watering of the eyes and running nose. Cocaine can produce a short-lasting psychotic illness, with marked paranoid ideation and hallucinations. Criminal acts may be carried out during such an episode.

Hallucinogenic drugs

Drugs of this type are taken mainly for the alterations they produce in the taker's perception of reality. Physical dependence does not occur, but users may greatly over-value the experiences induced by the drug.

LSD-25 (Lysergic acid dietylamide)

This is a synthetic drug which is taken for its ability to produce an hallucinatory state. It is effective in extremely small doses; if taken regularly tolerance rapidly develops, but is equally lost if the drug is discontinued. In its illicit forms the dosage is very variable, and hence its effects on an individual are difficult to predict. The drug starts to act within thirty minutes of ingestion, physical changes usually preceding the mental ones. These include a rise in blood pressure and pulse rate, slight rise in temperature and dilation of the pupils.

The mood changes may be either anxiety or euphoria, or alternation between the two. The most striking experiences are those of perceptual change. These may occur in all the sense modalities, but are usually particularly vivid in the visual field, and include illusions and hallucinations. Stimuli in one sensation may give rise to impressions in another sense, so that sounds are 'seen' or flashing lights are 'heard'. The subject's image of his own body may be affected so that he no longer feels he 'owns' his own body, or he may feel able to perform impossible acts such as flying.

Self control is lessened and aspects of the personality normally inhibited may be allowed free expression. Explosive outbursts of rage may occur.

Much has been written about the 'flashback' phenomena that happens in about 5% of people taking LSD. The mechanism of these episodes remains uncertain. They may consist of the sudden recurrence of an image experienced under the influence of the LSD, or a return of sensory distortion or hallucinations.

Some users develop a persistent hallucinosis, in which the images are sometimes horrifying and may give rise to considerable anxiety.

Cannabis (Hashish, Marihuana)

Though classified as an hallucinogenic drug, cannabis rarely produces hallucinations except when taken in the more potent forms. The question as to whether or not cannabis can produce serious psychological disorders remains unanswered. It would seem that if it does so, then it does so relatively rarely, and then in individuals who are predisposed to the development of such states.

The drug is normally taken to produce a mild degree of transient intoxication, in the same way that alcohol is used socially. The first effects are usually a feeling of lightheadedness and a sensation as of floating. The subject experiences a sense of relaxation and mild euphoria. There may be overactivity and talkativeness, the subject being of the opinion that his conversation is brilliant, witty and enlightening, while the observer may regard it as diffuse, rambling and banal. The user may experience a distortion of his time sense, usually feeling that everything has slowed down.

In higher doses the drug may give rise to much more marked emotional changes. These are sometimes ecstatic, but more often feelings of acute anxiety, terror and puzzlement. There may be pronounced feelings of depersonalisation or of derealisation. The subject may experience visual illusions in which colours take on a new vividness, or the shapes of objects become distorted. Visual hallucinations may occur, often of simple geometric forms, but sometimes of complex visions.

Frequent heavy use of the drug may give rise to tolerance and to withdrawal symptoms if the drug is stopped. Psychological dependence is much more common than physical dependence.

There is no specific 'cannabis psychosis'; a range of psychotic disorders have been described, which seem to have been triggered off by the drug and have spontaneously remitted when the drug has been withdrawn. Probably the commonest reaction is one of acute anxiety, which may lead to hysterical states in which the sufferer wanders about in a daze and has no recollection of events later. Acute paranoid reactions also occur with persecutory delusions and hallucinations. These usually remit as the drug wears off, but may sometimes herald in a persistent schizophrenic illness. Chronic personality changes in habitual users have been described, as have signs of organic impairment. The evidence for these states being due exclusively to cannabis remains uncertain at present.

Glue sniffing

A wide range of synthetic substances have been inhaled by those in search of intoxication, and the activity would be more accurately described as 'solvent sniffing'. However, adhesives have proved to be the most popular agents, perhaps because of their availability and relative cheapness—they are also easy to steal. The effects and risk vary depending upon which solvent is present in the substance inhaled. The immediate effects 'vary from inebriation to transient overt psychotic behaviour and psychoto-mimetic reaction; the results depend not only upon the intensity of exposure, but also on previous emotional and physical experience and the premorbid personality' [4]. Marked tolerance may develop, and some users show withdrawal symptoms if deprived of the drug.

Glue sniffing is not confined to children, but it is commonest among young males with a mean age of about thirteen years. It is usually a group activity, and correlates closely with poor scholastic performance and high truancy rates. Other associated factors are parental alcoholism, separation, deviant behaviour of siblings and lower socio-economic status.

References

Alcohol and drug abuse

Alcohol
1 Howard, et al. Camberwell Magistrates Court
2 Goodwin, D W, Crane, J B and Guze, S B (1969) Alcoholic blackouts—a review and clinical study of 100 alcoholics. *American Journal of Psychiatry*, **126**(2), 191–198
3 Goodwin, D W, Crane, J B and Guze, S B (1969) Phenomenological aspects of the alcoholic blackout. *British Journal of Psychiatry*, **115**, 1033–1038

Further reading

Riddick, L and Luke, J L (1977) Alcohol-associated deaths in the District of Columbia. *Journal of Forensic Sciences*, **46**, 493–502

Gerson, L W and Preston, D A (1979) Alcohol consumption and the incidence of violent crime. *Journal of Studies on Alcohol*, **40**, 3, 307

Gerson, L W (1978) Alcohol related acts of violence. *Journal of Studies on Alcohol*, **39**, 1294–1296

Edwards, G, Kyle, E and Nicholls, P (1977) Alcoholics admitted to four hospitals in England. Criminal records. *Journal of Studies on Alcohol*, **39**, 1648

References

Glue sniffing

4   Hayden, J W, Peterson, R G and Bruchner, J V (1977) Toxicology of toluene. *Clinical Toxicology*, **ii** (5), 549–559

5   Gibson, C (1968) Glue sniffing. *Canadian Pharmaceutical Journal*, **ii**, 207

6   Watson, J M (1977) Glue sniffing in profile. *The Practitioner*, **218**, 255

16. Psychopathic Personality

Psychopathy—the psychopath

The concept of psychopathy or psychopathic personality has been attacked on a number of grounds, and it has most certainly been the source of considerable confusion. Yet if it were to be banished by decree it would be necessary to invent some similar concept to replace it.

The confusion is in part the result of the way in which the concept evolved historically, in part because of the way in which the label became incorporated in legal statutes, and finally because the term is used so loosely as to have become almost synonymous with repeated criminality. The history of the concept is itself far from clear. Etymologically the word means 'derangement of the mind' and could thus be applied to any form of mental disorder, as is its derivative 'psychopathology'. It has come, however, to have a quite specific meaning.

When mental disorder came within the province of medicine and attempts at classification were made, it became apparent that most of the phenomena exhibited by the insane were also to be found in normal people, with the possible exceptions of delusions and hallucinations. For a time, it was considered that a diagnosis of true madness could not be made in the absence of these symptoms. Yet it was apparent that many people differed from normal in the degree to which they exhibited certain emotional reactions, such as grief or joy.

James Prichard writing in 1835 [1] referred to conditions of:

'madness consisting in a morbid perversion of the natural feelings, affections, inclinations, temper, habits, *moral dispositions*, and natural impulses, without any remarkable disorder or defect in the interest or knowing and reasoning faculties, and particularly without any insane illusions or hallucinations'.

He called these conditions moral insanity. Moral at that time had several different meanings and in the passage quoted it is used in the ordinary current sense of having to do with right and wrong. In Prichard's time, however, it was also used to mean roughly what is now meant by 'psychological.' Judging by the cases Prichard described as fitting into this category of moral insanity, it would seem that it was in this sense of psychological or emotional that he was using it in describing moral insanity. Subsequent writers, however, seem to have used that phrase to discuss cases in which the major disturbance occurred in the area of moral behaviour.

In 1891 Koch [2] tried to resolve some of the resulting confusion by suggesting that moral insanity be replaced by the term 'constitutional psychopathic inferiority'. This covered a wide range of conditions including neurotics, personality disorders and social deviations. This broad usage of the word psychopathy continued in the writings of German psychiatrists including Schneider (1934) [3].

In 1964 Cleckley [4] provided detailed clinical accounts of psychopaths and their behaviour. He stressed, however, that the behaviour was secondary to certain personality characteristics. These characteristics did not necessarily lead to anti-social or criminal behaviour. They could be expressed in many different ways and the particular form might depend on a range of factors such as intelligence, social class, education and social opportunity.

By concentrating on the central or primary personality traits, it is possible to distinguish between the psychopath and the criminal, whereas if behaviour is taken as the criterion no such distinction can be made. This is the fundamental error which led to the American adoption of the term sociopath in place of psychopath. To describe someone as sociopathic is to say nothing about the person, but only about his reaction to the particular society in which he finds himself. The psychopath having certain characteristic personality traits will remain the same in whatever society he finds himself, even though the response to his behaviour may be very different.

The particular traits which comprise the psychopathic personality are not exclusive to psychopaths, they exist to some degree in most people. The psychopath differs only in the extent to which they are present. There is no clear cut-off point and many individuals will fall into a grey area where one can argue whether or not they justify the label. A small number of people show so marked a degree of the characteristics that few would disagree that they justify inclusion.

Various attempts have been made to define the essential personality characteristics of the psychopath and there is a reasonable degree of agreement as to the important features which must be present, though they are expressed in various ways.

Primary features

(1)   An impaired ability to feel love and affection for others
This is an emotional inability not an intellectual one. The individual
may be well aware of how he should feel but cannot experience the
actual emotion. He may be extremely distressed by his inability to do
so. In many cases this inability seems to arise from lack of opportunity
to develop 'love' in early childhood, or from the repeated experiences of
rejection by those who should have provided love during the early
years.

(2)   An inability to delay gratification of needs
The normally developing child gradually learns to accept delay in
achieving his immediate wishes. Initially this delay may be imposed by
the parents until such time as they decide it is appropriate to respond
(by feeding, changing, etc.). Gradually the child learns that by
restraining his demands he not only gets what he desires, but the bonus
of approval and love from his parents. In the psychopath, this process
seems not to have occurred, so that when he feels a need he escalates his
demands until he obtains his wish. This inability to delay gratification
leads to impulsive behaviour without consideration of the long-term
consequences. It also leads to the psychopath having difficulty in
tolerating frustration.

Secondary features

(3)   A lack of feeling for others and a powerful need for instant gratification can lead to explosive acts of violence or aggression when his
wishes are frustrated.

(4)   A lack of feeling for others and a lack of concern regarding their
feelings for him produces an absence of guilt or remorse for what he
may have done.

(5)   Inability to delay gratification tends to lead to the pursuit of
short-term goals rather than those requiring persistence and effort.

(6)   Punishment of any kind when imposed by a loved person implies
the withdrawal of love by that person at least temporarily. This feeling
may be considerably more painful than the actual punishment, and acts
as a powerful source of reinforcement. Such reinforcement may not

occur in psychopaths. When there is any delay between the 'crime' and the punishment, they seem to be unable to associate the two together, and may then use the present punishment to justify further crimes. Whatever the underlying psychological or physical reasons they often seem unable to learn from experience or respond to punishment.

(7)   Lack of feeling and the need for instant gratification, plus the fear of ultimate rejection may lead to relationships being kept at a superficial level, with a tendency to exploit the other person rather than to be truly emotionally involved.

These aspects of the personality are only some of the factors which go to make up each unique individual. They will modify and be modified by other personality traits, and this interplay, combined with all the other environmental influences which occur, determines how the individual will express his potential. Attempts to classify 'psychopaths' into subgroups suffer from the same problems as all other attempts to put human beings into pigeon-holes. The classification which seems to have been most widely accepted is that of Henderson [5] who divided them into three broad groups:

(a)   The predominantly aggressive
(b)   The predominantly inadequate
(c)   The predominantly creative.

Members of both the first two groups may come into conflict with the law, while the last may be revered by society—particularly after their death.

In trying to establish the diagnosis of psychopathic personality, attention must be paid to the primary features as expressed by the individual and by examining aspects of the history which illustrate these traits. It is not sufficient to base the diagnosis on a history of criminality. Not all criminals are psychopaths and not all psychopaths are criminals.

The areas for consideration and the likely findings are as follows:

Early history

In a high percentage of cases there is history of a disturbed relationship with one or both parents during the early years of the child's life. This disturbance may have been due to the absence of one or other parent in physical terms, or the inability of a parent to relate normally to the child because of the parent's own psychological problems. In many instances, there is a history of active rejection by the parent, sometimes accompanied by actual physical abuse.

Paradoxically, in some cases the history is of extreme over-indulgence by the parents so that the child came to expect and demand instant satisfaction.

Education

The educational achievements of the psychopath frequently fall short of the potential suggested by his IQ. There may be evidence of academic success in those subjects for which he had natural ability, with abysmally low standards in those in which there was need for steady application. Schooling may have been disrupted by truancy or by bad behaviour leading to exclusion from class.

Work

There is likely to be a pattern of frequent changes of job, the change often being made on impulse and either for some short-term advantage, or as a result of disputes with workmates or superiors. In some cases, the picture is of apparent success at work until the individual impulsively destroys everything he has achieved.

Relationships

The inability to trust other people sufficiently to invest real love or affection in them tends to lead to superficial and transient relationships. There is often a characteristic and repetitive pattern for testing out behaviour. Expecting eventual rejection, the psychopath cannot resist provoking those around him to the point where they fulfil his expectations.

In sexual relationships there is often a history of promiscuity, which may be associated with a history of venereal disease. There may be a history of homosexual activity, though this does not necessarily imply a basically homosexual orientation. It may reflect a lack of immediately available heterosexual partners or it may be done for financial gain. In some cases, there may be a history of various sexual perversions.

Marriage is usually a stormy relationship with frequent partings and reconciliations. There may be evidence of physical violence towards the partner or children. Marriage is often entered into at a young age with subsequent divorce. Pregnancy is often a factor in the decision to get married. The marriage has often been strongly opposed by both sets of parents—a fact which merely encourages the pair to go ahead with it.

Drugs and alcohol

There may be a history of drug usage and drug abuse. Alcohol may be similarly abused. A relatively common pattern is that of episodic over-indulgence followed by periods of total or relative abstinence until the next 'bender'. Drugs may also be used in an episodic fashion, and involvement may be more in terms of pushing than using.

Violence

The combination of low tolerance for frustration, the wish for instant gratification and lack of concern for the feeling and well-being of others, provides an explosive mixture which may erupt into violence with relatively little provocation. Thus the history may contain many episodes of aggressive and violent behaviour, some of which may have resulted in criminal charges. Many such episodes will have been directed at members of his family and may thus have not come to official notice. In the more severely disturbed personalities where there is marked lack of feeling, the violence may be characterised by a degree of excessive savagery. In those who also have sexual deviations, the violence may be associated with sexual acts. In many instances, the violence is only directed at those who are relatively unable to defend themselves. Violence frequently occurs when the individual's already fragile control has been further diminished by drugs or alcohol.

Crime

The personality characteristics already described are likely to predispose the person to committing crimes if environmental factors combine to present an opportunity. In some instances, the crimes share certain characteristic features. They may be impulsive and poorly planned, and the possible rewards seem hardly commensurate with the likely punishment. Even well planned crimes often lack sensible plans for the disposal of the loot and the avoidance of eventual capture. The crime itself may be used as an excuse for an orgy of violence towards other people or directed at objects. The excitement of the act may be as important as the actual spoils.

It is necessary to repeat that criminality and psychopathy are not synonymous. Not all psychopaths are criminals and most criminals are not psychopaths.

The failure to distinguish between psychopathy and criminality has rendered much of the research into the subject relatively valueless. Many studies fail to state the criteria used in selecting the psychopath population, and when it is stated, it often amounts to no more than a history of repetitive criminal acts.

Studies of intelligence in psychopaths have almost all been carried out on those lodged in some form of penal institution or mental hospital. The majority of these investigations show a similar distribution of IQ as that found in the normal population. This may mean that psychopaths in general are more intelligent than normal as the institutional population is skewed as a result of the more dull ones tending to get caught.

Many attempts have been made to lend apparent scientific respectability to the personality traits derived from clinical observation by the use of objective personality tests.

The Minnesota Multiphasic Personality Inventory has been used and gives a personality profile on psychopaths which shows high scores on the Pd and Ma scales (Pd = Psychopathic Deviate, Ma = Hypomania scale). The profile pattern was described by Dahlstrom and Welsh (1960) [6] as delineating people who 'tend to be over-active and impulsive, irresponsible and untrustworthy, shallow and superficial in their relationships'.

Eysenk suggested that psychopaths could be distinguished by their scores on the Eysenk Personality Inventory, on which they should score highly on both the neurotic and extraversion scale. However, a number of investigations failed to support this theory. Eysenk [7] then modified the theory applying it only to actively anti-social criminals, lacking conscience or guilt feelings and excluding the introverted, withdrawn, inadequate criminals, who are also found in populations of recidivists. He postulated a third factor, psychoticism, in which there is a continuum from normal to psychotic. A person with a high P score is characterised by (1) being solitary, not caring for other people, (2) being troublesome, not fitting in, (3) being cruel, inhuman, (4) a lack of feeling, (5) being sensation seeking, (6) being hostile to others, aggressive, (7) a liking for odd things, (8) a disregard for danger, being foolhardy, (9) a liking for making fools of people, upsetting them.

These characteristics are much more the clinical description of psychopathy than psychotic, but when the questionnaire was given to the psychotic patients and to prisoners, the prisoners scored as highly as the psychotic non-offenders.

Eysenk has hypothesised that extroversion is an expression of an underlying predisposition of the nervous system to rapidly develop cortical inhibitory potentials. This leads to the individual acquiring conditioned responses slowly and extinguishing them rapidly. Thus Eysenk sees the psychopaths lack of socialisation as being an aspect of his poor capacity for conditiong.

Hare (1970) [8] summarised experimental investigations in psychopaths. These showed differences between 'psychopaths' and 'normals' in cortical studies, autonomic functions, learning performance and arousal.

1. Cortical studies

An underlying physiological disorder has been postulated for psychopathy and a variety of investigations carried out to try and elucidate this aspect. EEG studies have shown that a substantial number of psychopaths have abnormal traces. The most common finding is of widespread slow wave activity resembling the traces found in normal children. This has led to the theory that psychopathy is a reflection of cortical immaturity.

In about 10% of psychopaths the EEG shows evidence of localised abnormalities especially in the temporal lobes.

2. Autonomic nervous functions

A number of studies have demonstrated that psychopaths have a relatively low level of autonomic activity as measured by skin conductance and cardiac activity when at rest. Their response to stressful stimuli also seems to be more limited and the return to normal levels more rapid when the stress terminates.

3. Learning studies

Many studies have been done to investigate a range of learning processes in psychopaths. In general it would seem that they do not readily develop conditioned responses to fear-provoking stimuli. In general their ability to learn tasks that are not dependent on acquired fear is the same as the normal population.

4. Arousal

It has been suggested that 'psychopathy is related to a lowered state of cortical arousal with a chronic need for stimulation'. This idea to some extent relates to Eysenk's personality theories in which his dimension of extroversion is associated with a low level of cortical arousal while introversion is associated with a high level.

Legal Aspects of Psychopathy

In the Mental Deficiency Act of 1913 'moral imbeciles' were defined as:

> 'Persons who from an early age display some permanent mental defect coupled with strong, vicious or criminal propensities on which punishment has had little or no deterrent effect.'

Provision was made for such people who committed crimes to be sent to institutions for the sub-normal rather than to prison. This provision did not apply to people of normal intelligence, nor did it apply in cases of murder. The defence in such cases remains a plea of insanity under the McNaughton Rules.

The first opportunity for the Courts to take into account psychopathic personality without mental subnormality came with the passing of the 1957 Homicide Act:

> 'Where a person kills or is a party to a killing of another, he shall not be convicted of murder if he was suffering from such abnormality of mind (whether arising from a condition of arrested or retarded development of mind or any inherent causes or induced by disease or injury) as substantially impaired his mental responsibility for his acts and omissions in doing or being a party to the killing. Where the Court agrees that a killer at the time of his crime was in such a state of mind it must convict him of manslaughter and not murder.'

In the 1959 Mental Health Act psychopathic disorder was defined as:

> 'A persistent disorder or disability of mind (whether or not including subnormality of intelligence) which results in abnormally aggressive or seriously irresponsible conduct on the part of the patient and requires or is susceptible to medical treatment.'

Psychopathic disorder was one of the four categories subsumed in the Act under the general title of Mental Disorder, and the provisions for compulsory admission and treatment apply to it with certain limitations. Section 26, which allows for the detention in hospital of a patient for 1 year for treatment, could only be applied in cases of psychopathy under the age of 21 and would not be continued after the age of 25 without special permission. All patients so detained have the right of appeal to a Mental Health Review Tribunal, to appeal against the original order, its renewal, or its continuation past the age of 25.

Psychopaths who come before the Courts charged with a crime may have a Hospital Order made under the 1959 Mental Health Act on the grounds of their personality disorder. The provisions are stated in Section 60 and Section 65 of the Mental Health Act and are equally applicable to a person suffering from any other form of mental disorder.

The Order can be made by a Magistrates' Court if the offence for which he is convicted is punishable on summary conviction with imprisonment. Magistrates may make an order without convicting the person if they are satisfied that he is suffering from mental illness or severe subnormality but not psychopathic personality or subnormality. Before an order can be made under Section 60 the Court must have before it written or oral evidence from two medical practitioners at least one of whom must be approved under Section 28 of the Mental Health Act 1959. Both doctors must agree as to the form of mental disorder from which the defendant is suffering. They must also agree that the mental disorder is of a nature or degree which warrants the detention of the patient in a hospital for medical treatment, or the reception of the patient into guardianship.

The Court must then satisfy itself that:

'having regard to all the circumstances including the nature of the offence and the character and antecedents of the offender and to the other available methods of dealing with him, that the most suitable method of disposing of the case is by means of an order under this section'.

Such an order 'shall not be made under this section unless the Court is satisfied that arrangements have been made for the admission of the offender to the hospital specified in the order and that his admission will occur within 28 days of the making of the order'.

Section 65 allows a higher court to impose special restrictions on the discharge of an offender placed on a Hospital Order.

To invoke these provisions the Court must have had oral evidence from one of the doctors making the recommendation. The restrictions which apply under this section are that the power to grant leave of absence, to transfer, and to discharge the patient are rested solely on the Secretary of State. Patients who are allowed leave can also be recalled at any time by the order of the Secretary of State. The patient cannot appeal directly to a local Mental Health Tribunal, but has corresponding rights of appeal to the Secretary of State.

It is evident from the above that in many cases the possibility exists that an offender made the subject of a Section 65 order may be detained for periods far in excess of any penal sentence which might have been passed had his mental state not been taken into consideration. When capital punishment was in force, the plea of diminished responsibility on the grounds of psychopathic personality was an attractive alternative, but with the end of capital punishment, many killers would prefer to chance a definite period of imprisonment to the possibility of indeterminate detention in a special hospital.

This applies even more forcibly to those charged with less serious offences where a Hospital Order may seem appropriate, taking all circumstances into account and where the potential dangerousness of the offender makes Section 65 advisable. In some instances, the evidence of such dangerousness is not admissible in relation to the present charge and the offence itself may be relatively trivial, but the overall history is strongly suggestive that a serious offence will occur in the future.

References

Psychopathic personality

1   Prichard, J C (1835) *A Treatise on Insanity*. Sherwood, Gilbert & Piper, London
2   Koch, I L A (1889) *Leitfäden der Psychiatrie*. Ravensburg Dorn
3   Schneider, K (1934) *Die Psychopathischen Persönlichkeiten*. F. Deut, Leipzig
4   Cleckley, H M (1964) *The Mask of Sanity*, 4th edition. C U Mosky Co., St Louis
5   Henderson, Sir David (1956) Psychiatric evidence in court. *British Medical Journal*, **208**, 4983
6   Dahlstrom, W M and Welsh, G S (1960) *An MMPI Handbook*. University of Minnesota Press
7   Eysenk, H J (1964) *Crime and Personality*. Methuen, London
8   Hare, R D (1970) *Psychopathy, Theory and Research*. J Wiley, Snr., New York

Further reading

Craft M (1966) *Psychopathic Disorders and Their Assessment*. Pergamon Press, Oxford

17. The Ganser Syndrome

In 1897 Ganser [1] described what he called 'an unusual hysterical confusional state'. This had occurred in three prisoners who developed short lasting symptoms. These were, clouding of consciousness, hallucinations, and a peculiar response to questions which was described as giving 'approximate answers'. There was subsequent amnesia for the period of the disorder, recovery was otherwise complete and occurred abruptly.

Since his original description there has been considerable debate as to the nature of the syndrome, about its aetiology, and its relationship to other mental disorders.

The syndrome has largely been regarded as a manifestation of hysteria, but many of the reported cases have been associated with organic brain disease or functional psychosis. The syndrome has been described as occurring in schizophrenia, depression, general paralysis of the insane, alcoholic psychosis and following head injury. Not all writers have restricted the use of the term to cases in which there is definite evidence of clouding of consciousness, and seem to base the diagnosis mainly on the presence of 'approximate answers'. This has led to problems in differentiating between Ganser syndrome and hysterical pseudodementia (either hysterical or pseudo must be regarded as tautological in this title). A further area of debate is the relationship of the Ganser syndrome to prison psychosis. At the present time the occurrence of a Ganser syndrome in prisoners is quite rare, indeed cases in which all the symptoms originally described by Ganser occur seem to be extremely rare.

Scott (1965) [2] suggested that the Ganser syndrome should be differentiated from Ganser symptoms, the former being very rare but the latter relatively common. The syndrome should be restricted to cases where there is clouding of consciousness, approximate answers, abrupt recovery and amnesia from the illness. Hysterical pseudodementia would be restricted to cases with no clouding and where the apparent 'dementia' is occurring in a person of limited intelligence at a time of emotional stress.

References

Ganser syndrome

1 Ganser, S (1898) Über einen eigenartigen hysterischen Dämmerzustand. *Archiv für Psychiatrie (Berlin)*, **30**, 633–640
2 Scott, P D (1965) The Ganser syndrome. *British Journal of Criminology*, 5, 127–134

Further reading

Whitlock, F A (1967) The Ganser syndrome. *British Journal of Psychiatry*, **113**, 19–29

18. Sexual Deviation

The word deviation is not entirely satisfactory in this context. At various times in different societies almost all forms of sexual activity have been proscribed. Some activities may form a transient episode in normal sexual maturation and only be regarded as deviant if they persist, or are excessive in degree. However, at any given time certain acts are illegal and if indulged in, may bring the participant before the Courts. Sexual activity is usually regarded as deviant if it does not lead to heterosexual intercourse, is regularly performed in preference to intercourse, or has a compulsive component.

Paedophilia

In paedophilia the specific sexual attraction and preference is for partners who are physically immature. The term covers a wide range of behaviour in which an adult indulges in some sort of erotic activity with a child. Although not exclusively a male activity, it is vastly more common in men. The child may be of the same or opposite sex as the offender and may in some cases play an active role in provoking the offence. In the majority of cases this sexual activity consists of fondling, petting and genital manipulation and only rarely involves any attempt at vaginal or anal intercourse. There have been various attempts to classify paedophiliacs, one approach being to consider homosexual and heterosexual paedophiliacs separately. The vast majority are fixed in their sexual preference, but about 10% are bisexual in their orientation. Homosexual paedophiliacs have a somewhat higher rate of recidivism.

Mohr and Turner in a study of paedophiliacs in Toronto were able to demonstrate that based on the age of the offender, they could be divided into three groups with rather different underlying motives.

(1) The adolescent heterosexual paedophiliac could be regarded as showing retardation of normal psychosexual and social

maturation. The adolescent homosexual paedophiliac often had a history of adolescent exploitation, low intelligence, lack of social skills and poor social maturation.

(2) The middle aged heterosexual paedophiliac frequently shows a regression from adult sexual relationship to marital disharmony and social maladjustment. Alcoholism is frequently a significant factor. The middle-aged homosexual paedophiliac almost always shows a pattern of disturbed family relationships, with a dominating mother and an unsatisfactory relationship with father. Such men often see themselves in a pseudo parental role with their 'young friends' and lack insight into their own activities.

(3) Elderly paedophiliacs. In this group loneliness, social isolation and worry over impotence seem to be common factors. The relationship is often based on a need for affection rather than sex and there is a low incidence of recidivism in this group.

Victims

The role of the victims in paedophilia has been subject to a number of studies. Gibbens [1] has pointed to different patterns of child involvement and has suggested three types of interaction suggesting that the child/parent relationship determines both the offence and the reaction to it.

(1) Accidental victims—where the assault is a sexual offence usually committed by a stranger and reported at once to the parents. The vast majority come from stable homes—the child is well adjusted and they tend to get over the incident very quickly.

(2) Participant victims where it is part of a wide maladjustment. Children tend to come from problem families. The offence is only a slight addition to the many stresses of life.

(3) Participant victims where the offence represents a fairly specific disturbance—children are described as being rather precocious, sexually seductive, make immediate superficial relationships. There is no gross social disorganisation in the parents but a tendency to be over-concerned in the prettiness and seductiveness of their children. In the latter two groups current feelings about sexual activities seem to be grossly increased by criminal procedure.

In the United States it has been estimated that about 10% of all child abuse is sexual abuse. Follow-up studies of these children indicate that provided the court ordeal is not too great, the great majority settle and have no further problems.

Heterosexual paedophilia

It is possible to distinguish between men who show a persistent sexual interest in young (usually pre-pubertal) children and those whose paedophilia is situational in origin. The persistent paedophile is usually unmarried and may be sexually inadequate with adult women. They may indulge in a range of sexual activities from fondling of the genitalia to rape. The victim may be a relative or neighbour, or totally unknown to the offender. Unlike the situational offender, persistent paedophiles do not have a higher than average incidence of alcoholism.

Homosexual paedophilia

Some men are exclusively sexually orientated towards young boys. They do not in general have homosexual relationships with adult males. They rarely have satisfactory sexual relationships with women, though many enjoy platonic friendships with women and prefer female company. Some are, however, married and may have children of their own.

Those who indulge in less serious sexual assaults such as fondling or mutual masturbation may relate very easily to children in general. They may be very successful teachers, scout masters, or boys' club leaders. Some develop an obsession about small boys' penises and feel compelled to take any opportunity of seeing small boys in the nude. This may lead to a compulsive urge to touch the child's genitals and this may lead to a court appearance. Such 'acting out' may be precipitated by situational factors such as intoxication.

Some paedophiles have 'love affairs' in which they develop an overwhelming passion for a particular child. The relationship may become very emotionally intense and sexual activity may or may not occur.

The majority of paedophiles are aware that their sexual urges are both legally and morally wrong. They may struggle very hard to control themselves, but sometimes having 'given way' they indulge in an orgy of paedophiliac activity.

Secondary (symptomatic) paedophilia

Unlike those in whom the sexual drive is primarily directed towards children, there are many offenders in whom sexual abuse of children is merely one facet of their disorder. Many such offenders fall into the category of the impulsive psychopath. Such a man may respond to any opportunity that presents itself for any form of sexual activity. Having committed an impulsive offence he may decide to destroy the evidence against him and kill his victim—not from a sexual motive but to cover his tracks.

Paedophilia is sometimes associated with mental handicap. This may reflect a failure on the part of the offender to realise that his acts are illegal, but more often it arises because of the offender's difficulty in establishing normal adult sexual relationships.

Psychotic disorders may lead to child molestation as a result of hallucinatory instructions or delusional ideas.

Occasionally, hypomanics commit sexual offences with children. This may start as ordinary playing, but the excited hypomanic becomes sexually aroused and acts out in a disinhibited fashion.

A wide range of organic brain disorders may give rise to secondary paedophilia. Alcoholism is sometimes a factor. Any of the dementing disorders may lead to failure of control or lack of judgement. It is difficult to know whether child molesting only occurs in dementia in people who had a previous suppressed interest in such activities or whether it can occur in anyone.

Homosexuality in males

Since the 1967 Sexual Offences Act it is no longer a crime for a man to commit gross indecency or buggery with another man providing that both are over the age of 21, both parties agree, and the acts are done in private—that is without any other person being present, and not in a public lavatory. (Members of the Armed Forces are still subject to the special provisions of the Armed Services Act.)

The passing of this Act enabled many practising homosexuals to feel free from the threat of exposure and blackmail. Now that the majority of male homosexuals are not in danger of prosecution very few seek treatment in the hope of changing their sexual orientation. The majority now referred to psychiatrists are those whose sexual drive is directed at minors or those who persistently solicit or importune in a public place. Relatively rarely homosexuals with sadistic tendencies are referred as a result of some violent crime.

Every man has the potential for homosexual behaviour, but only some of those who indulge in homosexual acts are exclusively homosexual in their erotic orientation. Those who are exclusively or predominantly attracted to other men fall roughly into two groups, the effeminate, and the highly masculine. The former are the least numerous, but as they tend to flaunt their sexuality they are often regarded as 'typical' of homosexuals. They often 'cross dress', but have no wish to change their biological sex, nor do they cross dress for relief of psychic tension.

The highly masculine homosexual on the other hand may display no special features except for a lack of erotic interest in females. Not all are unmarried, some entering into such a relationship in order to disguise the true nature of their sexual interests.

In most large towns there is a homosexual sub-culture, often notable for its lack of class distinction. There are usually public houses, clubs and other social venues which are more or less exclusively patronised by homosexuals. Within this sub-culture a special jargon developed which gradually passed into common parlance. The 'gay' sub-culture may seem exciting to some young men who are not essentially homosexually orientated and they may be drawn into homosexual activity. Some will become exclusively homosexual, while others will change to heterosexual relationships at some stage.

The cause of homosexuality remains uncertain, but it is almost certainly multifactorial. There is a higher incidence of late birth order and high maternal age among homosexuals than among heterosexuals. Twin studies show that for identical twins there is an 80% chance of both being homosexual as compared to 10% for non-identical twins.

A wide range of childhood experiences have been postulated as causative of this condition.

Masochism

Masochism is obtaining sexual satisfaction by being hurt or humiliated by the sexual partner. The name derives from L. von Sacher Masoch (1836–1895) who wrote a number of novels in which the man submits to cruel and domineering women.

Masochists do not enjoy pain and humiliation in an indiscriminate way. They only derive pleasure from situations in which they have arranged to suffer, and in which *they* determine the type and degree of pain and mortification. Such people are, however, likely to find themselves in situations in which they lose control and may then end up as victims of their partners' sadistic drives.

Masochistic drives are not incompatible with ordinary sexual relationships. Indeed the compulsive masochist probably derives a relief from tension through his masochistic acts as well as sexual pleasure. There are often obsessional compulsive features to the behaviour with a very stereotyped pattern of activities.

The compulsive masochist differs from the psychopathic masochist who is solely concerned in sexual arousal as a result of pain, and who, when aroused, wants to achieve orgasm through intercourse or other sexual acts. Such men may be impotent unless aroused in this way. They not infrequently have sadistic tendencies as well.

In women mild masochistic traits are often part of a hysterical personality. Sometimes they are used to overcome a feeling of guilt about sexual activity. The woman who submits to bondage or corporal punishment or pseudo-rape can justify her enjoyment on the basis that she was the helpless victim and therefore not morally responsible. The relatively rare woman who can only respond sexually to physical pain has probably acquired this response as a result of previous sexual experience with a sadistic male.

Sadism

The sadist derives sexual pleasure from hurting, humiliating or tormenting his partner. The name derives from the Marquis de Sade (1740–1814) who wrote novels depicting acts of sexual cruelty. The sexual sadist may or may not be sadistic in his general non-sexual relationships with people. He is usually unable to form warm loving relationships with women. There are often other features of an obsessional personality. The homosexual sadist seems to be even more dangerous than the heterosexual. The compulsive sadist may feel constantly under pressure to act out his fantasies, or he may experience periodic episodes in which the compulsion to do so reaches an overwhelming intensity. Many can obtain satisfaction from acting out their fantasies in a 'theatrical' manner, paying a prostitute to simulate pain and suffering. Like the compulsive masochist the compulsive sadist may feel great shame and guilt about his activities and may struggle hard to control his impulses.

The sadistic psychopath, however, does not experience such feelings of guilt, and makes little effort to control his actions. In such individuals the sexual aggression is usually only part of a continuum of aggressive and violent behaviour.

Necrophilia

In necrophilia the sexual drive is directed at someone already dead. The perpetrator may dig up a body for the purpose, or more usually he obtains employment in a mortuary or funeral parlour. Many such offenders are psychotically ill or mentally handicapped, but cases are seen in which the deviation seems to exist in pure culture. In some instances the necrophiliac kills in order to provide himself with a corpse.

Sexual killings

Although there may be a degree of overlap between the motives leading to sexually linked killings, it is possible to separate out the following categories:

(1)   Killing following an illicit sexual act, either in panic, or in order to destroy a witness to the crime.
(2)   Killing for 'sexual kicks'—the psychopath who is surfeited with all other forms of sexual activities may kill as a form of diversion.
(3)   Sadistic sexual killing—killing as part of inflicting pain and suffering which is itself sexually arousing.
(4)   Killing in order to procure a corpse for necrophilic practices.

Fetishism

In this condition sexual arousal and satisfaction is obtained by collecting and/or handling inanimate objects. The objects usually chosen are those which have some indirect sexual association with women—underwear, shoes, stockings and the like. Such arousal by association is so common in males as to be regarded as normal; it only becomes a fetish when the object is totally substituted for the real person.

The condition can be divided into compulsive and situational fetishism.

Compulsive fetishism

The compulsive fetishist is an inveterate collector of his particular object. The desire to obtain it may reach a degree of craving comparable to that of an addict for his drug. The object obtained rarely seems to be new or unused. Secondhand articles may be satisfactory, but in many cases the object has to be seen in the possession of its owner and then stolen. It is this aspect which leads to the fetishist coming before the Court.

Symptomatic fetishism

In these cases, unlike the compulsive fetishist, the man is interested in having normal sexual relationships but finds that he is impotent in the absence of the fetish object. Thus he may only be able to manage intercourse if his partner is wearing black stockings, a plastic mackintosh, or whatever.

Transvestism

This is the act of cross dressing—the wearing of clothes appropriate to the opposite sex. As with the other sexual deviations it can be divided into compulsive and symptomatic forms.

Compulsive cross dressing

Most such men lead outwardly normal lives. They are not homosexual and are usually married and have children. They can perform sexually without difficulty though they may have a relatively low sex drive. From time to time they feel an intense need to dress up in female clothing. This desire may be strongly resisted and may lead to excessive drinking in an attempt to control it. When the compulsion is yielded to, the transvestite usually experiences a great relief of tension and it may be that this is the aim of the exercise, rather than sexual satisfaction. However, some compulsive transvestites masturbate when cross dressed. Some derive satisfaction from passing themselves off as females while others like to be recognised. Transvestites of this kind have no wish to change their sex.

Symptomatic cross dressing

Cross dressing may form part of both male and female homosexuality and may be the regular mode of dress adopted. It may also occur in transexuals. Transexuals are people who are repelled by their 'given' sexuality and wish to become a member of the opposite sex. When a transexual cross dresses he does not see it as an act of disguise, but an expression of his 'true' self.

Cross dressing in public by a man is not of itself a crime, unless as a consequence of the type of clothing worn, he indecently exposes himself. However, men dressed as women are often arrested on the suspicion that they are homosexuals and that they are 'soliciting or importuning in a public place for immoral purposes'. They may also be charged with 'insulting behaviour likely to cause a breach of the peace'.

Voyeurism

The vast majority of normal men and women are sexually aroused by witnessing the erotic activities of others. Sexual curiosity is part of the normal process of growing up. Some relatively immature individuals seek out opportunities to spy on people undressing or indulging in sexual activity. They may make a nuisance of themselves but are rarely dangerous.

The compulsive voyeur shows features of an obsessional disorder. He may resist the desire to peep, or may derive excitement from endlessly planning and rehearsing his system of spying. He derives sexual satisfaction from what he sees and may masturbate at the time. Most voyeurs are not dangerous but a small minority go on to more aggressive sexual crimes.

Treatment of sexual disorders

Many people with sexual deviations only seek treatment when faced with some form of legal punishment. Their motivation to change may be very poor, and this influences the likely outcome of treatment. Psychotherapy in all its forms has been used to treat almost all forms of sexual deviance. Results in general have been poor. In cases of exhibitionism it is difficult to compare results unless it is known whether first or subsequent offenders are being treated. In the case of first offenders, 90% are likely not to re-offend, whether treated or not, while repeated offenders seem to be little influenced by any form of treatment.

Behavioural methods have claimed some promising results and have the advantage of being relatively quick. Aversion methods have been employed in cases of homosexuality, fetishism, transvestism [2], exhibitionism [3] and paedophilia [4]. Such techniques are best combined with desensitisation of anxiety about alternative forms of sexual activity, and general help in social skills.

Drug treatment in the past has consisted mainly of giving oestrogens to males to damp down their sexual drive. The use of these drugs has been limited by their feminising side effects. More recently cyproterone acetate (Androcur) has been used to reduce deviant sexual behaviour without totally abolishing socially acceptable sexual drive [5]. The use of such agents raises a number of ethical and legal questions.

References

Sexual deviation

1 Gibbens, T C N and Prince, J (1963) *Child Victims of Sex Offences*. Institute for Study & Treatment of Delinquency
2 Marks, I M and Geldor, M G (1967) Transvestism, fetishism, etc. *British Journal of Psychiatry*, **113,** 711–730
3 Evans, D R (1967) An exploratory study in the treatment of exhibitionism. *Canadian Psychology*, **8,** 162
4 Marshall, W L (1973) The modification of sexual fantasies. *Behavioural Responses and Therapy*, **11,** 557–564
5 Bancroft, J and Bancroft, H J (1975) The control of deviant sexual behaviour by drugs. *Journal of International Medical Research*, **3,** Suppl. 4

Further reading

Bancroft, J (1974) *Deviant Sexual Behaviour; Modification and Assessment.* Clarendon Press, Oxford

Part 4 The Role of the Psychiatrist

19. The Examination and Court Report

In general the examination and formulation of a report in a legal case is the same as an examination in ordinary clinical practice, and a competent general psychiatrist is perfectly able to give a competent forensic report. A few significant differences should be borne in mind.

1. The referral

In clinical practice the vast majority of referrals will be made by the patient's family doctor, with occasional referrals from consultant colleagues, social services departments and the like. In forensic work the vast majority of referrals will come from defending solicitors. Some will be referred by other doctors, by probation officers, court officials, or even the Home Office. Defendants may be referred for psychiatric reports at any stage of the case. The referral may be concerned with fitness to plead, with the possibility of insanity as a defence, or in order to determine the most appropriate sentence if he is found guilty. The source of referral may influence the offender's response to the psychiatrist—if asked by the defence, the offender may regard the psychiatrist as an ally, while if asked by the prosecution, he may regard him as an enemy.

The whole question of the role of an expert witness is debatable. It has been suggested that the expert should indulge in advocacy—that is, trying to make out the best possible case for 'his' side, short of distorting the facts. However, in Britain, it is usually considered that the expert witness should attempt to be neutral and keep a balance between those aspects of the evidence that favour the defendant and those that do not.

Essentially, the role of the psychiatrist is to assist the Court by his special knowledge. It is not his task to tell the Court what to do, nor to offer advice that is outside his special expertise.

The source of referral is very important in terms of the relationship to the accused. When introducing yourself to the client you should start by making it completely clear who has asked you to see him. The purpose of the interview should be explained to him and he should be advised that your opinion may be given in Court. He should be told that he is under no obligation to answer any questions if he chooses not to.

2. The interview

The interview should be conducted in a setting where strict confidentiality can be observed. In many prisons the facilities provided are far from satisfactory—and if so, this fact should be recorded in the report.

The value of the initial interview will be directly proportional to the amount of preparation done by the psychiatrist and those involved in preparing the case. The psychiatrist should have a clear idea as to the purpose of the examination, particularly with regard to whether there is any question as to fitness to plead. Much valuable time will be saved if there is an accurate social history available—this may have been taken by a probation officer, solicitor's clerk, or private detective. Do not, however, assume that it is accurate.

Each statement in the report should be checked with the client and modified as necessary. This process is still much quicker than trying to extract raw material for oneself. It also tends to highlight gaps and omissions, and in filling these in significant material sometimes emerges.

The psychiatrist should have details of the present charges, and past convictions. He should also have copies of any statements made by the defendant, and by witnesses if available. These should have been studied in advance, and points needing further discussion noted.

The interview should rarely last for more than an hour to an hour and a half, as at this point mutual fatigue sets in. It is much better to finish fresh and return another time.

During the interview, detailed notes should be made, recording significant comments verbatim. The date, time and place should be recorded on the notes. It is important to record any gestures, mannerisms or special behaviour. A brief note about the offender's general physical appearance may be helpful.

At some stage in the interview, the details of the alleged crime should be discussed. While in law the assumption is of innocence until guilt is proved, in medicine it is often necessary to assume guilt until innocence can be established (every lump in the breast is malignant until proved otherwise). In cases where in spite of all evidence to the contrary the defendant insists on his innocence, the value of the psychiatric report is limited, as it is obviously impossible to explore the reasons for the act if the act is itself denied. In discussing the accusation and the statements a good deal can, however, be gleaned about the defendant's general attitudes and reactions.

A full history of previous illnesses should be taken and, if relevant, note made of hospital admission dates so that if required case notes may be obtained for study. Particular attention should be paid to any neurological disorders including significant head injury. Epilepsy should always be enquired about, including a family history of this disorder.

Previous mental disorder should also be asked about in simple everyday terms—'have you suffered from your nerves; do you get low spirited; have you ever been treated for nerves or admitted to a mental hospital?' Again any referrals for psychiatric opinion or treatment should be noted and details obtained from the appropriate source.

A detailed assessment of the present mental state is made in the ordinary clinical way, and on the basis of this assessment a decision reached as to what, if any, special investigations are required. Laymen are always disproportionately impressed by apparently objective scientific tests as compared to clinical judgement (so, regrettably, are many doctors). Where there is some question of the level of the defendant's IQ it is best to have it properly tested by a competent clinical psychologist. Personality tests rarely seem to add to a properly taken clinical history, and projective tests such as the Rorschach are more useful as a source of court-room humour than scientific clarity.

Having completed the examination, it may be necessary to interview other people who know the defendant, just as one would interview relatives in the ordinary clinical situation. When the defendant is remanded in custody, it is often helpful to ask the opinions of those who are looking after him. This is particularly true when he is remanded in the hospital wing of the prison. The warders will often have had previous psychiatric nursing experience, plus long acquaintance with criminals. Their judgement is often sound and they have the advantage of long periods of contact with the prisoner. While someone can 'act mad' for short periods, it is very difficult to keep it up day in day out in the presence of skilled observers.

Having examined the client as many times as is felt necessary and obtained all relevant information including the results of special investigations, it is necessary to prepare a report for the Court. In doing this it should be constantly remembered that it is to be read by laymen.

Write in simple English and avoid jargon as far as possible. If a technical term has to be used, define it as accurately as possible. Be concise—the amount of paper work associated with a case is frightening and there is no value in adding to it unnecessarily. Lawyers have a conventional way of preparing and setting out their documents and it is helpful if the psychiatrist adopts their technique for his report.

3. The report

1. The report should open with a statement of the psychiatrist's full name, qualifications and present appointment. If appropriate, it should include the statement 'I am approved under Section 28 of the Mental Health Act 1959'.
2. Where and when and in whose presence (if anyone) the interview was conducted.
3. Relevant documents which have been examined before or after the examination should be listed. Failure or refusal to produce such documents on someone's part should also be noted.
4. Family and Personal History of the Defendant
It is not usually necessary to set this out in great detail, particularly if the information is available to the Court in a social report. It is important to select and emphasise those aspects which are relevant in arriving at a diagnosis, or which may be important in determining appropriate disposal.
5. The Account of the Crime given by the Accused
This aspect of the report will depend on whether the defendant is pleading guilty or not guilty and it may involve accounts of episodes with which he is not currently charged. It is advisable to discuss this with the solicitor and if necessary write it on an addenda to the main report which can be submitted, if appropriate, after the verdict has been arrived at. It is legitimate to comment on his present attitude to the crime if he admits to it, such as his degree of remorse, his attitude to any likely punishment and his views regarding his future behaviour.
6. Ancillary Behaviour
Though not directly involved in the events leading up to the crime, certain aspects of behaviour may be relevant in establishing the context. The defendant's use or abuse of alcohol or other drugs on a regular or intermittent basis may be important. The manner in which he usually relates to other people, and the ways in which he deals with

frustration may be relevant. An assessment of his general level of social competence may be included in this section.

7.   Present Mental State

This should be described in adequate detail so that if disputed by another expert witness, the respective barristers can ask useful questions. A statement of the salient positive features is sufficient. It is not necessary to list an endless string of negative findings. At the end of the description there should be a statement of the general diagnosis in the terms used in the Mental Health Act—i.e. 'this man is suffering from mental illness, or subnormality of intelligence, or psychopathic personality.' This can then be followed by a more specific diagnosis, though it is important to remember that the Court is not interested in academic debates about whether the illness is schizophrenia or manic depressive psychosis, it is merely concerned to know whether or not he has a mental illness.

8.   Mental State at the time of the Crime

This must obviously always be a matter of some speculation, yet it is the vital aspect as far as the mental state may be adduced from descriptions given by witnesses at the time or shortly after, including police witnesses. The nature of the crime itself may give some indication, though it is dangerous to assume that because the crime was crazy so was the perpetrator. The nature of the diagnosis is of crucial importance in assessing the likely mental state at the time. In cases of chronic organic brain disease, the mental state is not likely to have been very different than at the time of examination unless there was evidence of a super-added confusional state. Chronic schizophrenia which has not remitted for some long time is also unlikely to differ substantially. Depressive states are much more difficult to assess. It is to be expected that many people facing a criminal charge will be depressed as a result of that fact and objective evidence must be sought as to whether or not the depression predated the event leading to the prosecution. The greatest problem is presented by disorders which are essentially episodic such as epilepsy, unless the nature of the crime itself suggests an inexplicable and short-lasting episode of disordered behaviour.

9.   Relationship of Mental State to Criminal Responsibility

Even in cases where it can be shown conclusively that at the time of committing the offence the person was suffering from some form of mental disorder, this of itself need not be relevant. In each case it is necessary to determine to what extent the sufferer was able to form the necessary intent to commit the crime, or to determine to what extent his ability to refrain from committing it was impaired. A clear statement of opinion on this matter is a vital part of the report, as this is an area where lawyers will attempt to obtain over-simplified answers.

10.   Fitness to Plead

In all cases referred for psychiatric opinion, it is worth considering the question of fitness to plead and including an opinion in the report, however unnecessary it may seem. Inevitably, the one time it is omitted, someone will raise it at some stage of the trial. Rather than the bald statement—this man is fit to plead—state the criteria, saying whether or not each is satisfied. Fitness to plead is, of course, a variable state and it may be necessary to re-examine the defendant just prior to his appearing in Court.

11.   Management

Essentially, it is the task of the psychiatrist to advise medical treatment if he feels it to be appropriate and not to offer advice on any other form of disposal. However, it would seem legitimate to extend this to commenting on the possible effects on the defendant of alternative forms of punishment if such effects can be clearly predicted from his mental state and past history. In order to make useful suggestions, the psychiatrist must be aware of what possibilities exist both within the medical services and the penal system. In cases where hospital treatment is recommended, he should advise the Court if a suitable place is available and if it is not, he should state the reasons why placement is not possible.

A very important aspect in deciding on the appropriate management is an assessment of the 'dangerousness' of the offender. This is discussed later.

Giving evidence in court

Many psychiatrists avoid forensic cases because they fear appearing in Court. As a result of watching television dramas in which the expert witness suddenly confesses that he, in fact, was the murderer, they anticipate that at best they will be made to look foolish and at worst they will get six months for contempt of court. The reality is a great deal less alarming. At first the strange surroundings and unaccustomed formalities may provoke anxiety, but this soon diminishes. Simpson [1] pointed out that there are four essentials in dealing successfully with giving evidence: (1) preparation, (2) clear exposition, (3) limiting oneself to one's field of competence, (4) tolerance and courtesy.

Preparation

The expert witness will be allowed to refer during his evidence to his records and original notes in the case, and he should be sure that he takes these with him into the witness box, having divested himself of all other encumbrances. He should have familiarised himself with the contents of the documents to the point where they need only be referred to as an aide-mémoire. The notes, if copious, should be properly organised and readily accessible so that the Court is spared endless turning of pages and the undignified scrabbling about when the whole lot break free of their fastenings and drift down onto the Court officials below.

The witness should have thought through his evidence and antici-pated likely questions, if necessary looking up relevant parts in the literature or consulting with more experienced colleagues. However, it is important to remember that it is not the purpose of the expert witness to lecture the Court. He is there to assist in arriving at a judgement not to demonstrate his knowledge.

Prior discussion with Counsel can be invaluable. Lawyers and psychiatrists suffer the disadvantages of a shared language which creates the confusing impression that they mean the same things when they use the same words. Legal language in relation to mental events came to a halt some time in the nineteenth century and it can be difficult to translate these terms into contemporary psychiatric jargon. Much of the mutual misunderstandings which arise are due to semantic confusion. Time spent attempting to clarify what Counsel wants to know and what the psychiatrist is able to say can save much wasted effort in the box.

Clear exposition

The art of communicating involves marshalling the relevant informa-tion into a logical sequence, expressing it in simple, unambiguous language and delivering it in an audible clear voice. In addition, the non-verbal communication by the witness may create as much, if not more of an impression than the spoken word. Court hearings are serious formalised rituals designed to elucidate the truth. A witness who gives the impression of being himself, seriously concerned with the matter in hand will create a better impression than one who seems to regard the proceedings with disdain or levity. Courts are by their nature conservative and have certain stereotype images of what professional men should look and sound like. This may be reactionary and regrettable, or sound and desirable, depending on one's point of view, but should be taken into account. A witness who fidgets, shuffles, looks away, slouches, scratches himself or yawns is likely to be less convincing than one who stands straight, looks directly at the judge or jury and shows interest in the questions asked.

When asked a question, there is no hurry to answer it. Time taken to consider the question and its implication is time well spent. The shorter and more simple the answer, compatible with doing justice to the question, the better. Do not elaborate on the answer, unless you specifically wish to be asked a following question. If you do not know the answer to a question say so—if no one knows the answer say that also. When alternative opinions are put, often backed by reference to some eminent authority, allow the existence of different views, but if you consider your own opinion valid, stick to it.

When directly addressing the judicial head of the Court use the correct mode of address:

A Coroner is called 'Sir'
A Magistrate 'Your Worship'
A Crown Court Judge 'Your Honour'
A High Court Judge 'My Lord'.

Restricting oneself to one's field of competence

Possibly because psychiatry contains so many areas of uncertainty, psychiatrists are particularly prone to making ex cathedra statements on almost any topic other than their own speciality. Such temptations should be strictly resisted in court. Invitations to speculate on hypothetical matters above and beyond the facts of the case should be politely declined. Equally, however, attempts to denigrate one's own experience and expertise by describing it as 'pure guesswork' should also be rejected.

Tolerance and courtesy

All the professionals involved in a trial have a specific task and will be trying to perform that task to the best of their ability. The job of the defending Counsel is at least to sow seeds of reasonable doubt in the mind of Judge or jury as to the veracity of the prosecution case. The task of the prosecuting Counsel is the precise opposite. Both are bound by strict rules of evidence and procedure, but within these rules they are entitled to exploit any technique for casting doubt on their opponent's case. The evidence of the expert witness is liable to the same scrutiny as any other. The witness should not regard attacks on his evidence as being a personal affront. He should not be upset by the use of emotive words to give a different shade of meaning to what he has said, but should patiently insist on his own version if it more accurately conveys his meaning. Medical experts usually start with a considerable advantage in that most lawyers have only a layman's knowledge of the subject, albeit usually a highly intelligent layman's interest. Thus most lawyers when cross-questioning medical witnesses, and particularly psychiatrists, feel at a disadvantage. It is tactically unsound to try and increase this uncertainty by being patronising or pompous, as both are liable to provoke a desire to puncture the bubble, and in verbal exchanges the lawyer is likely to win hands down. Polite and courteous responses to questions, however irritating they may be, always proves the most effective tactic.

Recommendations for disposal

The psychiatrist must always remember that the decisions as to the disposal of an offender are made by the Court and the Court is entitled to totally disregard any advice offered it by the expert witness. In practice, great consideration is given to any such recommendations and the Court is often only too glad to be offered some alternative to imprisonment. The doctor must also remember that his recommendations should be restricted to advise on possible treatment. It is not his business to recommend hanging or transportation, whatever personal views he may have on the subject. The options open to him can be listed as:

For prisoners who are for sentencing.

(1) No treatment at all
(2) Out-patient treatment on a voluntary basis
(3) Out-patient treatment as a condition of probation
     (The offender has to agree to any such condition)
(4) In-patient care on a voluntary basis
(5) In-patient care as a condition of probation
(6) In-patient care in ordinary mental hospital on a compulsory Hospital Order under Section 60 of the 1959 Mental Health Act

(7) In-patient care in ordinary hospital without ~~restriction~~ limit as to time of detention. Hospital Order Section 65 (1959 Mental Health Act)

(8) In-patient care in special hospital offering special degree of security. Hospital Order Section 60 (1959 Mental Health Act)

(9) In-patient care in special hospital without limit as to time (Section 65, 1959 Mental Health Act)

(10) Psychiatric treatment in prison

(11) Psychiatric treatment in a psychiatric prison.

The last two are purely recommendations and are not binding upon the prison psychiatric service.

Prior to trial, a variety of recommendations can be made:

(1) Remand to psychiatric unit for assessment
(2) Transfer to psychiatric hospital for treatment
(3) Remand in custody for psychiatric reports
(4) Transfer from prison to hospital under Section 73 (1959 Mental Health Act).

In making a recommendation, the doctor should state what he feels is appropriate and should not be influenced by outside pressures to say something else. Should it not be possible to implement his recommendation, he should state the reasons for this and if necessary offer some other less satisfactory suggestions. It should be made clear that these are less satisfactory and represent a compromise.

In making a recommendation for a Hospital Order it is as well to remember that if the offender is subsequently found not to be susceptible to treatment, or not in need of treatment, he cannot then be transferred to prison and so early discharge may result. On the other hand, an offender sentenced to prison, subsequently found to need treatment, can be transferred to a hospital for as long as is required and can then return to prison to complete his sentence. Thus in cases of doubt and where public safety requires a long period of detention, it may be better that in the first instance the offender be dealt with in the penal system.

In the case of people found 'Not Guilty by Reason of Insanity' or 'under disability' (unfit to be tried), the Court *must* order that the accused be admitted to a hospital to be specified by the Home Secretary. In all other cases a court is not obliged to order hospital care or other medical treatment. The offender may be sent to prison irrespective of the nature or severity of his mental disorder. While in prison he may receive such psychiatric treatment as the prison medical service can provide.

It is generally agreed that offenders suffering from severe subnormality are not suitably placed in prison and should, if necessary, be placed in the care of the local authority, in suitable hospitals, or if needing special security, in one of the special hospitals.

The question of security is the most difficult problem in deciding on the management of the mentally disordered offender. The degree of security needed reflects the dangerousness of the offender, and that dangerousness includes danger to himself, danger to the staff looking after him and danger to the public at large and other patients in the hospital.

Over recent years the trend has been to open all the locked wards within the mental hospital and to allow free egress for both patients and visitors. Many hospital wards have been integrated so that even separating male and female patients may be difficult if not impossible. Along with this has developed an unwillingness on the part of many working in hospital to accept even relatively slight risks of violence from the patients. Additionally, since the introduction of the major tranquillisers, the general level of violence within the mental hospital has greatly diminished. This in turn has led to a loss of expertise in dealing with such outbursts. These factors have led to a lowering of tolerance for disturbed behaviour and a rejection of patients who even a few years ago would have been regarded as perfectly containable in the ordinary ward setting. The suggested solution of establishing regional secure units has hardly got off the ground, and where they have, the cost of looking after patients in them has been astronomical.

Assessment of dangerousness

Determination of whether or not an individual is dangerous, is very difficult and it must be emphasised from the start that the ability of psychiatrists, or anyone else for that matter, to predict the likelihood of an individual carrying out dangerous behaviour is very low. Research on the prediction of future violence has not yet provided us with any predictive indices of either high reliability or validity. In none of the methods used has a prediction rate of higher than two wrong judgements for every one right judgement been achieved. In spite of this, the assessment of the degree of dangerousness is regarded as the most important task facing the forensic psychiatrist. It is certainly the most difficult.

The concept of dangerousness is an extremely diffuse one. Dangerousness in the broad sense is the threat that an individual poses to society in general or other individuals in particular. It is relative to the state of that society at the time and cannot, therefore, be defined in absolute terms. There are many forms of danger, both to people and to objects, concrete or abstract. We may speak of social danger, political danger and moral danger as well as physical danger. In all these, attention is being drawn to the fact that something is a potential risk, that it is attended with uncertainty, and that it is potentially unsafe. According to the situation pertaining at the time, the action of a given individual may be seen either as heroic and courageous or deviant and dangerous. In the context, however, of the forensic examination, dangerousness can be conceptualised as a propensity to cause serious physical injury or lasting psychological harm.

The setting in which the examination of the client is carried out also influences the procedure of the assessment of dangerousness. For example, the assessment of the dangerousness of an individual who has committed no offence and who presents in the course of routine out-patient clinic imposes very different problems from those of an individual who is before the Courts having already committed a serious crime. Similarly judgements affecting the release of people already deemed dangerous and detained in long term institutions pose other problems.

The psychiatrist should remember that other disciplines have an equally important contribution to make in the assessment procedure and that thoroughness of information collecting, interviewing and discussion with other relevant people (psychologists, social workers, family doctors, relatives, etc.) are essential if even a limited degree of prediction reliability is to be achieved.

The assessment of dangerousness, then, involves an attempt to balance those factors in the individual which may be considered as instigators to aggression as opposed to those factors which may be either positively or negatively related to inhibitions against aggression. MacDonald [2] writing on the assessment of dangerousness suggested three areas of importance:

(1) Factors relating to the offence and behaviour at the time
(2) Environmental factors
(3) Internal factors or specific characteristics of the offender.

Each of these areas should be considered in terms of their contribution to the balance between acting aggressively and controlling such actions.

Offence and offence behaviour

The nature of the offence itself is not predictive of future offence behaviour. Homicide is not necessarily a prediction of future dangerousness especially when it represents a solitary act of aggression. In a 26-year follow-up of criminal homicide parolees, Gernert [3] found that of 2,568 cases only 13 committed further homicide. Walker [4] has suggested that there is a relationship between the committing of serious offences and the likelihood of further serious aggression and it is suggested that offenders with a record of at least two offences of serious violence or sexual molestation should be given long preventive sentences, as he maintains there is a high probability of further such offences occurring.

The majority of sex offenders are not re-convicted (only about 15% being so) and some of these are for other non-sexual offences. Only some 2% of the convicted sex offenders are persistent and exclusive sex offenders.

Details of the offence

The events preceding it and the circumstances of the offence are all vitally important in any assessment process. Where possible police reports, social work reports and family reports should be obtained. As far as violent offences are concerned, it must be remembered that over 80% of violent offences are domestic offences and only a small minority of violent offences result in either serious or permanent injury to the victim. In sex offences too, particularly those involving children, a high percentage of victims are known to the offenders prior to the commission of the offence.

Environmental factors

Environmental factors are probably the least well understood but in the opinion of many authorities are also probably the most important in the lead up to any dangerous behaviour. Particular emphasis has been placed in recent years on the role of victims as instigators of offences, or at least as major contributors. The morbidly jealous man may not be dangerous until he forms a relationship with a woman who is herself sexually provocative with other men. The young man with a psychopathic personality and a drink problem may be of minimal dangerousness until he co-habits with a young woman who has small children by another man. The depressed man who kills his wife and children is then dangerous to no-one until he remarries, has a second family and becomes depressed again.

Apart from the victim, other environmental factors that should be considered are the place of the offender within the community and the environmental setting within which the individual lives. The pressures, both social and family, that may be put upon him, the particular stresses of his environment in terms of finance, relationships, work, etc., must be considered.

Most attempts to assess dangerousness have been based on factors operating within the individual. Kozol [5] describes those features of the personality which are usually described as forming the psychopathic constellation, impulsivity, inability to delay gratification and indifference to the suffering of others as being indicative of dangerousness. Impulse control is certainly an important factor and some assessment of this can either be obtained from psychological tests or from developmental history. Again it must be emphasised that it is often the combination of situational events and personality that are more important in an assessment than mere personality variables themselves. Thus the over-controlled individual who normally never uses violence may explode within the context of the given situation into severe and apparently bizarre destructive behaviour. Research has also shown that the inadequate psychopath is often more likely to commit seriously violent offences than the aggressive psychopath.

Attention should be paid to the individual's ability to handle stress and the techniques that he has used in the past to do so. Sometimes violence may provide forms of anxiety relief and on other occasions it may be part of a sado-masochistic personality. Brittain [6] has described some features to be looked for in the seriously sadistic personality.

Other factors that should be considered are intelligence, in terms of how well equipped the individual is to handle problems of his environment; possible organic factors including epilepsy; and the role, if any, of mental illness. Mental illness *per se* plays little part in dangerousness, the determining factors having to do far more with the personality. However, in those relatively rare cases where appropriate personality features are combined with a psychotic illness, the risk becomes much higher. One commonly described triad that is said to be associated with subsequent dangerous behaviour is the presence in childhood of cruelty to animals, fire setting and enuresis. These must be taken, however, as part of global indicators for disturbed early personality development rather than having any magical properties of their own.

The assessment of dangerousness, therefore, involves trying to weigh the relevant significance of these various factors. At present it is impossible to quantify these factors in a way which allows appropriate predictions to be made. However, both for the sake of the offender and his potential victim such predictions have to be attempted. If at the time of the examination a detailed report was made, it would facilitate future attempts to assess those features which have predictive value. In compiling such a report the following topics should be considered:

1.   *The attitude of the offender to the violence he used:*

   (a)   Was he angry at the time and if so with the victim, himself or some other person? Was the anger realistic, justified or unrealistic and disproportionate?

   (b)   Did he derive any pleasure or satisfaction from injuring his victim?

   (c)   Did he identify in any way with his victim?

   (d)   Is he self punishing or masochistic?

2.   *The attitude of the offender to himself:*

   (a)   What features in himself does he approve of, and of what is he critical?

   (b)   On whom does he model himself?

3.   *The attitude of the offender to other people:*

   (a)   Does he see them as potential victims or as potential exploiters?

   (b)   Does he see people as individuals or merely as objects to be exploited?

   (c)   Does he see people as separate unique individuals or merely as members of classes (e.g. women, blacks, peasants, etc.)?

4.   *How does he relate to others?*

   (a)   Is he socially isolated, or an involved member of a community?

   (b)   Is he socially skilful or inadequate?

   (c)   How does he relate to authority figures?

   (d)   How does he relate to those over whom he has some authority?

5.   *How did he relate to his family?*

   (a)   Is there a history of conflict with either or both parents?

   (b)   What was his relationship to his sister?

6. *What degree of impulse control has he demonstrated in the past?*

   (a) What sort of work record has he, and what were the reasons for changes of job?

   (b) How has he behaved in response to provocation?

   (c) What does he consider to be 'provocative behaviour'?

   (d) How does he respond now to provocation?

   (e) What techniques of control does he use?

7. *What are his social circumstances at present, and what will they be at the end of any sentence imposed?*

   (a) Are there any potential victims in his immediate environment?

   (b) Are such victims likely to be present in any future immediate environment?

8. *Was there any evidence of mental illness at the time of the offence?*

   (a) If psychotic at the time, what relationship, if any, did the illness have to the offence? In cases where the offence arose directly out of the psychosis, then the prediction of dangerousness is in part related to the prognosis of the illness.

9. *Is there any evidence of drug or alcohol abuse prior to or during the offence?*

The above is not intended as a check list for scoring 'dangerousness' as no specific weighting can be given to the various items. It merely ensures that no major aspect is ignored when considering the individual in question.

References

The examination and court report

1   Simpson, K (1967) *A Doctor's Guide to Court*, 2nd edition, page 51, Butterworth, London

Further reading

Bluglass, R (1979) *Medicine, Science and the Law*, **19**, 2, 121

Gradwohl, R (1979) *Legal Medicine*, 3rd edition. John Wright, Bristol

Bartholomew, A A (1962) The psychiatric report for the court. *The Criminal Law Review*, pp 19–32

Henderson, Sir David (1956) Psychiatric evidence in court. *British Medical Journal*, **208**, 4983

Home Office (1974) Mentally Disordered Offenders. (Information for Doctors on the Respective Roles of Hospitals, Local Authorities and Prison Services)

Assessment of dangerousness

2 MacDonald, J M (1969) *Psychiatry and the Criminal.* C C Thomas, Springfield, Illinois

3 Gernert, P J (1966) *A 20-year Comparison of Release and Recidivists.* Commonwealth of Pennsylvania Board of Parole

4 Walker, N et al (1970) *The Violent Offender; Reality or Illusion. Occasional Paper No. 1, Oxford Penal Research Unit.* Blackwell, Oxford

5 Kozol, H L et al (1972) The diagnosis and treatment of dangerousness. *Journal of Crime and Delinquency*, **18**, 371–392

6 Brittain, R P (1968) *Gradwohl's Legal Medicine* (Ed) F Camps. John Wright, Bristol

Parliamentary Acts

Index